The UNHysterectomy:
Solving Your Painful, Heavy Menstrual Bleeding Without Major Surgery

Holly Bridges

Foreword by Sony S. Singh, MD, Ob-Gyn

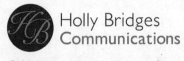
Holly Bridges
Communications
Delivering your message to your audience

First edition.

All rights reserved. No part of this publication may be reproduced or transmitted in any form or by any means, electronic or mechanical, including photocopying, recording or any information storage and retrieval system, without permission in writing from the publisher.

Published and distributed by

Holly Bridges Communications
1619 Orleans Blvd.
P.O. Box 58016 Orleans Garden
Ottawa, ON K1C 7E2

Tel: 613-863-0545
Email: holly@hollybridgescommunications.ca
www.hollybridgescommunications.ca

Contact us for information on author interviews, speaking engagements or bulk sales

Library and Archives Canada Cataloguing in Publication

Bridges, Holly, 1958-

The unhysterectomy : solving your painful, heavy bleeding without major surgery / Holly Bridges, author ;

Sony S. Singh, medical editor. – 1st ed.

Includes bibliographical references.
ISBN 978-0-9879360-0-4

1. Hysterectomy – Popular works.
2. Menorrhagia – Popular Works.
3. Generative organs, Female – Diseases – Popular works.
4. Surgery, Unnecessary – Popular works. I. Singh, Sony S., 1975- II. Title.

RG391.B74 2012   618.1'453   C2012-901308-0

The information and opinions expressed in this book are not a substitute for the advice of a physician. Only your doctor or a qualified health provider can provide you with advice and recommendations for your situation. This book presents information that has been researched and written by a patient for patients. Some of the testimonials contained herein are composites to protect the privacy of those interviewed. Medical experts have reviewed the medical information for accuracy; however, the information provided should not be used as the sole source of information regarding hysterectomy and its alternatives. Every attempt has been made to present a balanced account of this issue. Any errors or omissions are unintentional. Holly Bridges, her heirs, administrators, successors, agents and assigns, cannot be held liable for injury or damages resulting from use of the information provided in this publication.

Canadian edition. Each of the medical and surgical treatments described herein is also available in the United States. The author has not been paid to endorse any of the products or procedures identified in this book. Some names have been changed to protect the privacy of individuals.

Editor: Donna Dawson, CPE
Medical Editor: Sony S. Singh, MD, Ob-Gyn
Design: Patrick Mathieu, Philippe Faucher, d2k Communications
Printed and bound in Canada

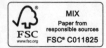

MIX
Paper from
responsible sources
FSC® C011825

For my beautiful daughters, Alex and Katie.
I love you to the moon and beyond.

"Be the change you want to see in the world."

– Mahatma Gandhi

Contents

Foreword

Sony S. Singh, MD, FRCSC (Ob-Gyn)

As a gynecologist and the Executive Director of the Canadian Society of Minimally Invasive Gynaecology, I applaud Holly for helping women understand that they have options when it comes to reproductive health matters such as abnormal uterine bleeding, fibroids and pelvic pain. Too long have we ignored the common problems of heavy menstrual bleeding and painful menses that affect our women of reproductive age. These women are our workforce, our caregivers, our teachers, mothers and sisters.

When the medical system fails to advocate on behalf of patients, it takes a special individual to lead the charge that will lead to change. Holly is that special individual. Her enthusiasm, hard work, dedication and ability to communicate have led to this moment. Through her book, website and social networking, I believe we will see a discussion that is nationwide and will lead to patient empowerment and physician accountability.

Lastly, I must comment on Holly's passion. To see results in any campaign, a clear vision and focus must be present. Holly has not wavered in the years I have known her from this single goal of assisting women in Canada. Through this commitment, I am certain we will see a significant impact on the way we discuss hysterectomy and alternatives to hysterectomy for women in Canada over the upcoming years.

About Dr. Singh

Dr. Sony S. Singh is Director of Minimally Invasive Gynecology at the Shirley E. Greenberg Women's Health Centre at the Ottawa Hospital. He is also an Assistant Professor with the University of Ottawa Department of Obstetrics and Gynecology. After completing his medical and residency training at the University of Western Ontario in 2005, he completed fellowships in advanced pelvic surgery at the University of Toronto and the University of Sydney from 2005 to 2007. Dr. Singh is the Executive Director of the Canadian Society of Minimally Invasive Gynecology.

Dr. Singh is world renowned for his surgical expertise in treating deep infiltrative endometriosis through minimally invasive means and is one of the leading experts in Canada in laparoscopic (keyhole) hysterectomy. He also specializes in minimally invasive alternatives to hysterectomy, such as hysteroscopic and laparoscopic myomectomy and hysteroscopic endometrial ablation. Dr. Singh has been instrumental in developing new guidelines for the treatment of abnormal uterine bleeding and endometriosis for the Society of Obstetricians and Gynecologists of Canada, guidelines which had not been updated since 2001.

Dr. Singh has also helped develop a new index known as *technicity* to measure the appropriateness of hysterectomies being performed in Canadian hospitals and to encourage gynecologists to perform the procedure less invasively, either vaginally or laparoscopically. Dr. Singh has achieved one of the highest technicity rates in the world.

He lives in Ottawa with his wife and their three children.

Acknowledgements

This book is the fulfillment of a lifelong dream and there are many people to thank for making this important project a reality. First, my beautiful daughters, Alex and Katie, for your love, patience and understanding while I wrote – you are my everything, now and forever; my husband, Gaston, without whom none of this would have been possible – I love you so much; my dad, a strong and spirited 92-year-old veteran of the Second World War, for teaching me tenacity and determination; my mom, whose love was unconditional to the end; my sister Lesley, for taking such good care of Dad and for sacrificing so much of her time to care for him; my beautiful sister Sue, who first raised that tiny seed of doubt in my mind, and whose spirit and laughter is with me still – I miss you every single day; my editor, Donna Dawson, for giving my words such tender loving care; Sarah Moore at *More Magazine* for first allowing me to share my story there in the September 2009 issue – the success of that article, and its subsequent pick-up in *Readers' Digest*, gave me the courage and the idea to write this book; Dr. Hassan Shenassa and Dr. Nicholas Leyland, for their kind and gracious support and for never saying no to my relentless, late-night emails despite their enormously heavy schedules; Dr. Jennifer Ashton for supporting a relatively unknown Canadian author and for sharing your time, expertise and re-tweets! Your support and mentorship have been an inspiration on so many levels; Mitch Joel, author of *Six Pixels of Separation*,[1] for unknowingly inspiring me to bypass traditional publishing and media channels to go it alone and create a living, breathing, multi-dimensional platform where women from around the world can

---

[1] Mitch Joel, *Six Pixels of Separation* (New York: Business Plus, 2009).

connect on this important issue; Janna and Steve at Marketing Breakthroughs for helping me crystallize my vision; Patrick, Daniel, Céline and Philippe at d2k for their incredible talent and support; my girlfriends, for their patience and understanding; and all the women, physicians, scientists and experts who took time out of their busy practices and schedules to be interviewed, especially those Canadian gynecologists and family physicians who went out on a limb and risked professional retribution by speaking out on this very important topic.

Finally, my thanks to Dr. Sony S. Singh at the Shirley E. Greenberg Women's Health Centre at the Ottawa Hospital, the medical editor of *The UNHysterectomy,* for the countless hours you have spent on this project. Working with you on this project has been the crowning achievement of my career and one of the highlights of my life. Your genius as a scientist and as a surgeon is surpassed only by your kindness, compassion and passion for helping women. When I first came to you in 2008, you opened a window on a world I never knew existed and gave me options I could barely pronounce, never mind have. What a powerful and empowering gift you are giving to women, not only through the extraordinary care you extend in your daily practice, but through this book. Thank you for never giving up on me, even though it took me three years to finally write this book. I only wish all women could see how hard you and your colleagues in minimally invasive gynecology are working on our behalf – between seeing patients, taking call, the OR, travelling to train other gynecologists in laparoscopy, attending and speaking at international conferences, pushing for change within our healthcare system, and revising surgical guidelines, all the while finding time to fulfill your roles as husbands, wives, mothers and fathers. Sony, I owe your wife and children a huge hug and a thank you for giving so much of their precious time with you to me. Their support has no measure.

It's curious – almost every woman I interviewed for this book who finally found a gynecologist who could help her without invasive surgery felt that somehow fate, or a higher power, played a hand in bringing them together. Looking back on it, I believe my sister Sue was watching over me that day and brought us together. What were the chances I would find you a mere three weeks after you had moved to Ottawa? I truly feel we were meant to meet so we could work together on this very important project. You are a rising star in the world of minimally invasive gynecology and I sincerely hope this book will bring you and your colleagues the recognition you deserve for what you are doing for Canadian women. It is an honour and a privilege to work with you.

PART I

INTRODUCTION

The Big Picture

Ladies, we have an opportunity on our hands, an opportunity to change the course of history in our country. Not by marching or carrying placards or burning effigies, but by simply saying these three words: *enough is enough*. If we make the kind of change I am proposing in this book, we could save the Canadian healthcare system almost a billion dollars over the next five years alone, free up our precious operating rooms for those who really need them and radically alter the way our society perceives and treats women's gynecological health. We may even increase our fertility rates as many younger women who were previously told hysterectomy was their only treatment option are now able to conceive and have children due to an explosion in technology that has the potential to one day make the need for hysterectomies almost obsolete. You will discover all of these treatments in this book and meet many of the women who have had them. (Sadly, most women are not being told about these options, which is one of the reasons I wrote this book.)

Hysterectomy hysteria

For generations, Canadian women have undergone hysterectomy, or as our sisters in Quebec call it, "la grande opération," one of the most life-changing operations we can ever have.

Hysterectomy is the most common major surgery performed on Canadian and American women, second only to Caesarean section. Many women are in disbelief when I share with them that 47,000 Canadian women underwent the procedure in 2008/09 while an average of 650,000 American women continue to have the surgery *every year*. Anywhere from 60 to 80 percent of all hysterectomies are elective and *medically unnecessary* (a controversial statement, as you will discover), chosen by women out of sheer desperation to treat a painful and debilitating medical condition that affects one in four women around the world.[2] In 2011, the Society of Obstetricians and Gynecologists of Canada (SOGC) introduced a new clinical term for the condition: heavy menstrual bleeding (HMB). This new designation is an important first step in increasing public awareness and understanding of this crippling condition that is far too often written off simply "a woman's problem." The condition is commonly referred to as abnormal uterine bleeding; I prefer to call it a bloody nightmare.

The majority of HMB cases are caused by benign growths called fibroids, which can grow in or on the lining of the uterus. For some unknown reason, they can cause tremendously heavy periods. As many as 80 percent of women have fibroids, but only about 25 percent experience any symptoms. Still, one out of four women suffers from these troublesome tumours. Some women experience symptoms of HMB when they are as young as 12 years old while others suffer closer to menopause. Women afflicted with pelvic pain and HMB suffer from serious, sometimes life-threatening anemia, take prescription pain killers to keep from doubling over in devastating pain, are rushed to hospital for emergency blood transfusions, lose thousands of dollars a year in lost wages and money for supplies, and have the same quality of life and level of function as heart attack and stroke victims entering rehabilitation.[3]

Yet these women are not in rehab or even in hospital. They are the women you see every day at work, on the soccer field, in the grocery store or on the bus, struggling to stay afloat while

---

[2] M. Zinger, "Epidemiology of Abnormal Uterine Bleeding," *Modern Management of Abnormal Uterine Bleeding* (London, UK: Informa Healthcare, 2008), 25.

[3] K. Frick, "Financial and Quality of Life Burden of Dysfunctional Uterine Bleeding among Women Agreeing to Obtain Surgical Treatment," *Women's Health Issues* 19, no. 1 (Jan-Feb 2009): 70-8.

their world is secretly crashing down around them because of the numbing exhaustion and crippling pain that are the signposts of this condition. Women with HMB are geniuses at hiding it. I know because I was one of them.

"Some women with chronic blood loss are constantly fatigued and always running low but unfortunately their body gets used to it so they may not think it's anything serious," says Dr. Catherine Allaire, a gynecologist in Vancouver and director of the University of British Columbia Women's Centre for Pelvic Pain and Endometriosis. She is also the director of education with the Canadian Society of Minimally Invasive Gynaecology (SMIG). "These women tend to have more subtle symptoms, like chronic fatigue, not being able to exercise very much, a heart rate that goes up too fast or heart palpitations, but mostly it's overwhelming fatigue. These kinds of subtle symptoms may not be something that takes them to the emergency room or even to their family doctor if they're highly tolerant of fatigue. As women, we have so many things going on that fatigue is a common symptom.

"I had always had heavy periods but in 1993 I was diagnosed with endometriosis. The bleeding and pain got so bad that in February I haemorrhaged for three days straight because of my fibroids. I would stand up and the blood would just fall out of me. One day I passed out in the shower. My son heard me fall and called his auntie to rush me to the hospital. They had to give me four blood transfusions to bring me back. They recommended a uterine artery embolization for me instead of a hysterectomy because it was less invasive. It's taken me a year to finally feel normal again. I can feel such a difference now."

– Sarah, 45

"But I have patients who are literally walking around with hemoglobins of 80 and I keep asking them how they are able to function. I [have to] convince them to do something about it and they are always reluctant. Women simply cannot continue living with hemoglobin of 80 without catching up with iron replacement. The risk of heart attack is too great. Maybe not for a 25-year-old, but if you're a woman in your 40s who is a bit overweight, has diabetes or who smokes, you're a sitting duck for other predisposing factors. So if you add the extra strain of anemia, it's the tipping point. You can go into pulmonary edema [a build-up of fluid in the air sacs of the lungs that can cause shortness of breath], you can have heart strain or in the worst-case scenario, you can have heart failure."

> **Anemia**
>
> *Anemia occurs when the red blood cell count, or hemoglobin, is less than normal because of chronic blood loss. Normal hemoglobin levels in women range from 115 to 155. Anything below 80 or 90 may require a red blood cell transfusion.*
>
> *– Thunder Bay Regional Health Sciences Centre*
> www.tbh.net

Suffering in silence

HMB is the number one reason women seek a hysterectomy in Canada, the US and around the world.[4,5] Although the numbers may seem high, the majority of women who suffer from HMB never seek treatment, choosing to suffer in silence, thinking their symptoms are just a normal part of being a woman. Women with endometriosis, perhaps the cruellest of all benign gynecological conditions (in which cells from the lining of the uterus grow in other areas of the body), suffer for an average of seven years in Canada before being properly diagnosed, if they are diagnosed at all.

And even if women with HMB are diagnosed, the nightmare of finding appropriate treatment, or waiting for a hysterectomy begins, adding months, if not a year or more, to their suffering. Wait

[4] G. Vilos for the Society of Obstetricians and Gynecologists of Canada, "Clinical Practice Guidelines: Guidelines for the Management of Abnormal Uterine Bleeding," *Journal of Obstetrics and Gynaecology Canada* 23, no. 8 (2001): 704-9.

[5] American College of Obstetricians and Gynecologists, "Management of Anovulatory Uterine Bleeding," Practice Bulletin no. 14 (March 2000).

times for hysterectomy in Canada vary from 12 weeks to 12 months or more, depending on the type and where a woman lives.[6] Sadly, wait times for minimally invasive alternatives to hysterectomy, which I will describe in this book, can be three to four times longer than for hysterectomies, for a variety of reasons.

As if the number of hysterectomies is not alarming enough, it's the manner in which they're performed that's the most astounding. Despite national guidelines set by SOGC suggesting that most hysterectomies should be performed either vaginally (where the uterus is removed through the vagina) or with the assistance of laparoscopes (which are inserted into the belly through tiny keyhole incisions), and despite decades of studies proving that laparoscopic-assisted hysterectomy is better for women, the majority of hysterectomies in Canada are still performed through deep, invasive cuts through the abdominal wall.[7] "Old habits die hard in gynecology," is how one researcher put it. A report in the November 2009 issue of the *Journal of Obstetrics and Gynaecology Canada* revealed that in 2008, 60 percent of the hysterectomies performed that year were done abdominally; in the United States, 66 percent of hysterectomies performed in 2003 were done the same way.

> *I had an abdominal hysterectomy about a year ago. While I don't regret my decision because my periods have stopped, it's difficult because I've gained 25 pounds that I just don't seem to be able to shake, and I still get PMS symptoms because they left my ovaries. So I feel like I'm getting my period but nothing happens. It's weird. I think the system could be a little more sensitive to women having hysterectomies. They put me in the maternity ward after my surgery and the day I got home a nurse from the public health unit called to congratulate me on my new baby. She obviously confused me with someone else. I was done having kids, but it was hard, you know?*
>
> – Melissa, 39, Ottawa

---

[6] Canadian Institute of Health Information, *Health Indicators 2010*, 18.

[7] P. Laberge and S. Singh, "Surgical Approach to Hysterectomy: Introducing the Concept of Technicity," *Journal of Obstetrics and Gynecology* 31 (Nov. 2009): 1050.

"Patients, gynecologists, and health care administrators all have a stake in improving outcomes, reducing morbidity and remaining fiscally responsible," say the study's authors. "Advocating for minimally invasive hysterectomy requires a strategy that clearly and simply outlines the benefits and risks of various approaches. One such strategy is known as technicity." *Technicity*, which I will explore later in this book, is a tool developed in France to measure the appropriateness of surgeries. Some chiefs of gynecology at Canadian hospitals are now applying technicity to determine whether women are receiving the appropriate care for their particular condition.

So what?

Minimally invasive surgery of any kind, not just for women, is simply safer, less intrusive and better for patients. It employs smaller, or no, incisions, carries a lower chance of infection and organ perforation and recovery time is much quicker.

In terms of minimally invasive gynecological surgery, whether we're talking about hysterectomy or not, there are cost savings to be had as well. Not including admission to hospital, six weeks to recover (in the case of an abdominal hysterectomy), time off work, lost wages, abdominal scarring, possible re-admission for complications, the risk of bladder or bowel perforation, nerve damage, incontinence, sexual dysfunction (and in the case of ovary removal, an increased risk for developing heart disease, lung cancer and osteoporosis), hysterectomies cost the Canadian healthcare system $192 million in 2008/09 in hospital admissions alone, not including surgical fees.[8] To put it crudely, *gynecologists earn more to remove a uterus than they do to leave one in.*

---

[8] Canadian Institute of Health Information, *Health Care in Canada* 2010, 33.

The average hysterectomy in Canada earns a gynecologist about $500, whereas an endometrial ablation (which removes only the lining of the uterus) or a myomectomy (removal of only the troublesome tissue) pays about $250. Surgical fees for gynecology are so outdated in this country that gynecologists actually earn *twice as much* for invasive abdominal hysterectomies as they do for less-invasive, uterus-sparing procedures – even though these procedures take two to three times longer to perform and require greater, more intricate, surgical skill.

"Unfortunately, some of the more invasive procedures actually pay better than some of the less invasive procedures," says Dr. Nicholas Leyland, President of the Canadian Society of Minimally Invasive Gynaecology and Professor and Chair of Obstetrics and Gynecology at McMaster University in Hamilton, Ontario.

"Take for example hysterectomy. If the amount a surgeon is paid for a hysterectomy is X dollars in Ontario, to do it laparoscopically it's X times 1.25. So you get 25 percent more for doing it, but in fact the majority of the time it takes to do this procedure laparoscopically [through keyhole incisions versus an abdominal incision] is significantly longer. So you are able to do fewer cases per unit time in a particular day in the OR. The other issue is you have a wait time. You've got patients waiting for a procedure. So if you eat up all your operating time, which is limited, with these longer cases, then your wait time is actually even longer for the other patients waiting. So it's a very complex issue. The reality of it is that most physicians who are doing this kind of surgery actually do take a cut in pay to be able to provide this kind of care for women."

Dr. Wendy Wolfman is an associate professor of obstetrics and gynecology at the University of Toronto and was named the 2009 North American Menopause Society practitioner of the year.

> I don't think remuneration is the major consideration [but it is a factor]. Currently a veterinarian receives more money than a gynecologist to do a hysterectomy. (I believe this says something about the current values of our society and the attitudes towards women's healthcare.). Most gynecologists receive more remuneration for a day in the office than a day in the operating room. I believe most gynecologists want to offer the very best care for their patients. Gynecologic surgeries are under-remunerated in the current schedule of benefits when compared to comparable services for men.

In Canada, doctors are paid only for the services they provide, not their overhead costs[9] whether they earn $2,500 per day in the operating room for five hysterectomies or $500 for two minimally invasive procedures. In essence, they're contractors. Additionally, with the pressure to reduce wait times for *all* surgeries inside the hospitals where they operate, gynecologists are asked by their hospital administrators to *justify* why they can put only two patients through the operating room in a day (with minimally invasive procedures) instead of four or five.

> If you paid gynecologists $1,000 more to perform a laparoscopic hysterectomy or a laparoscopic alternative to hysterectomy, guess how many more surgeons would do laparoscopic cases? If you paid surgeons $1,000 more to do an endometrial ablation rather than a hysterectomy, you'd have your hysterectomy rate go down and you'd have your ablation rate go up. If you gave people an incentive, say for every uterus you save, I'll give you an extra ten bucks, it would happen.
>
> – Anonymous gynecologist

---

[9] Herbert JMV Emery, Chris Auld and Mingshan Lu, *Paying for Physician Services in Canada: The Institutional, Historical and Policy Contexts* (Edmonton: Institute of Health Economics, 1999), 4.

"The number of hours it takes to do a laparoscopic surgery is maybe four hours instead of two or three. So if I have 20 people waiting for an operation and I only have one day every three weeks in the operating room and I use that time to only perform two surgeries instead of five, in a way I'm denying [surgery] to two or three additional patients who I could be operating on. It's about more than [trying to perform less invasive surgery]. It's about recognizing that we can't offer the service to all the women who are clamouring at our door," says Dr. Wolfman.

"The Ontario Society of Obstetrics and Gynaecology is trying to improve the situation and the fee schedule for gynecology because it's abysmal. I'm at the point I'm no longer frustrated. Now I just love what I do. I feel very blessed that I can look after women. For me, it's not about the money. I get a lot of satisfaction from looking after my patients and making them better."

Some provinces have begun to pay gynecologists an extra 25 percent for performing laparoscopic surgery but those increases have come after many years of lobbying. However, the lack of *substantive* incentives is a factor.

> **Did you know?**
>
> A minimally invasive surgical suite costs approximately $700,000. There are fewer than a handful of these suites in all of Canada.

There are, in fact, disincentives: some provinces have set up centres of excellence for bariatric surgery (a term used to describe a number of procedures that can help patients lose weight) to treat obesity (in most cases, a preventable condition). These centres are luring general surgeons away from their practices because of the bonuses being offered for bariatric procedures. Imagine if provincial health ministries set up centres of excellence in minimally invasive gynecology. Many gynecologists have told me they would flock to practice in such centres and train to perform laparoscopic procedures because the provinces would pay them incentives for doing so.

The push towards increasing access to laparoscopic surgery for women is slowly beginning to increase, especially in British Columbia, where hysterectomy rates are the lowest in the country. A recent study showed that if every province achieved BC's hysterectomy rate of 311 per 100,000 women age 20 or older, our healthcare system could save $19 million *every year*.[10]

"BC is greener than anywhere else in Canada in the sense that the culture is more natural and more conservative," says Dr. Allaire. "I find patients here are more interested in preserving their body parts and asking for the least invasive care possible. The atmosphere here is all about nature and being as natural as possible and not doing things that are perceived as unnatural, like taking a body part out.

> **Did you know?**
>
> *British Columbians have one of the longest life expectancies in the world and BC women gained an additional 3.2 years in life expectancy between 1990 and 2009?*
>
> *Hysterectomy rates in BC vary widely between regions, with the Northern Interior having the highest rate at 624 per 100,000 and Vancouver lowest at 162 per 100,000.*
>
> – "The Health and Well-Being of Women in British Columbia," 2008. www.gov.gc.ca

"But there are pockets. Vancouver probably has the lowest hysterectomy rate in BC but in other pockets like northern BC women want their uterus out. It's a different mentality. When these women come to see me, it's all I can do to convince them to have an ablation [see Chapter 13] instead of a hysterectomy. They say, 'I just want

---

[10] Canadian Institute of Health Information, *Health Indicators 2010*, ix.

the hysterectomy. I just want it out.' And so I'm doing the opposite, trying to talk them out of it." Personal preference and cultural bias are very real, and are two of the many factors which currently prevent our country from achieving the kind of savings described above. That and the fact that our healthcare system is built around putting people in hospitals rather than assigning the most appropriate care, be it in an operating room, outpatient clinic or doctor's office. But the system is in overdrive just trying to keep up, and who wants to be the one to call a time out? The public policy think tank the Fraser Institute did just that in its 2010 report *Value for Money from Health Insurance Systems in Canada and the OECD*. (The OECD is the Organisation for Economic Co-operation and Development.)

"The federal government should suspend enforcement of the *Canada Health Act* on a five-year trial basis in order to allow provinces to experiment with new health insurance policies such as patient cost-sharing, private competition and private medical insurance. Any chance of meaningful reform in Canadian health insurance is effectively hobbled by the outdated *Canada Health Act*, which forbids many of the successful policies used in other countries," said Mark Rovere, the institute's associate director of health policy research. "By taking a temporary 'time out' on enforcing the act, provincial governments would have the option to experiment with new policies without fear of financial penalties. The trial period would allow us to test different options to improve the delivery and accessibility of health care for ordinary Canadians by emulating the policies used in other countries."[11]

---

[11] Fraser Institute, *Value for Money from Health Insurance Systems in Canada and the OECD* (Vancouver: Fraser Institute, 2010), ix.

Wait times are a factor

Taking the leap suggested by the Fraser Institute, however noble, requires an entirely different approach to healthcare, and who can say how such a bold move would affect people waiting for surgery now? Unfortunately, wait times for gynecological surgery were not identified as a priority in the 2004 $41 billion federal Health Accord that promised to reduce wait times by 2014 in five priority areas – cancer, cardiac care, diagnostic imaging, joint replacement and sight restoration.[12] That leaves gynecologists to compete against their own colleagues for access to operating rooms, where the majority of gynecological procedures are still being done (rather than in outpatient clinics).

"Our healthcare system has to be open minded enough and our health policy experts have to understand that there are other options," says Dr. Leyland. He continues,

> And we're not talking about private medicine. We're talking about taking many of these activities that do not belong within hospitals and putting them into safe, publicly funded, freestanding areas where they can be provided in a less expensive environment. There are lots of situations where we can provide this kind of care in a much more fiscally responsible environment, to save money and to give women access to these technologies.

> There are lots of people across Canada who are very, very frustrated with the system. And they're beating their heads against the wall because they just don't have the skills or the understanding to figure out how to best change the system from within. And that's a pretty frustrating place to be – and they're also extremely busy clinicians. It's very difficult to find the time to do this additional kind of work when you're taking call and trying to look after patients on a day-to-day basis. So I think the problem really is getting enough people together with the skills and the interest to be able to advocate for women. We also need more women to help us.

---

[12] Health Canada, "A 10-Year Plan to Strengthen Health Care," Sept. 2004, www.hc-sc.gc.ca.

This has to come from a patient advocacy movement. It's not going to come from the medical profession because for too long I think we've been seen as being very self-serving and we're not the people who are going to provide the answers to these problems. I think the message has to come from patients, because they are the legitimate owners of our healthcare system.

In other words, we need to take HMB out of the bathroom and into the boardroom. When women have growths the size of footballs protruding from their bellies, or lesions on their vital organs that cause tremendous pain and bleeding, and are told to go back home because it's nothing more than their period, something is wrong.

> *You can hardly watch a sporting event without multiple men, or famous men, talking about how much better their erections are by taking the little blue pill. I think we need to start talking about heavy menstrual bleeding the same way. The problem has been kept in the shadows for far too long.*
>
> – Dr. Elizabeth Stewart, Mayo Clinic, Rochester, Minn.

Consider this: fibroids are the leading cause of hysterectomy in Canada and the US.[13] More women have hysterectomies for fibroids than for all gynecological cancers combined, according to Dr. Elizabeth Stewart, one of the world's leading experts on fibroids and author of *Uterine Fibroids. The Complete Guide*.[14] Yet due to an explosion in technology and state-of-the-art techniques, there are at least 10 minimally invasive treatments and procedures that could treat these benign tumours without hysterectomy. But they're not being utilized. No wonder anywhere from 60 to 90 percent of hysterectomies are elective. Most women choose to have them out of sheer desperation, begging for a permanent solution.

"I was done," is a statement I commonly hear from women with HMB. I ask you, at a time when the Canadian healthcare

---

[13] Toronto Endovascular Centre.
[14] E.A. Stewart, *Uterine Fibroids. The Complete Guide* (Baltimore: John Hopkins University Press, 2007).

system can ill afford to waste money on unnecessary surgeries and expensive hospital admissions, why are we not giving these women the support they need, even though we have gynecologists clamouring to perform these less-invasive procedures?

Why, when so many options exist, are the majority of doctors still advising us to remove our "private" parts?

Why, even though the *Canada Health Act*[15] ensures equal access to equal care for all Canadians, do rural women have a hysterectomy rate almost double that of women in urban areas?

Why, even with a proven connection between ovary removal and a twofold increase in our risk of developing heart disease and lung cancer (the leading cancer killer of women), are doctors still removing our ovaries as insurance against ovarian cancer?

And why, indeed, do we – the same generation of women who have the freedom, education and chutzpah to do and have whatever we want, be it fly fighter jets, conquer Mount Everest, research the cure for cancer or practically call in CSIS if we suspect someone has hurt our child – suddenly acquiesce and shrink into nothingness when our doctors open their mouths? I think I know why: because as Boomer women, we have one foot in the 1950s and 60s, when women put up and shut up, and the other foot in the 2000s, when women can do, be and say pretty much anything they want.

Sometimes I think we spend more time shopping for a pair of shoes than we do for a doctor. But if someone told me one of my daughters needed surgery, you can bet your stilettos I would stop at nothing until I found the best, most qualified, respected doctor who could perform the safest, most effective, least invasive procedure possible. My

---

[15] Justice Canada, *Canada Health Act*. www.laws-lois.justice.gc.ca/eng/acts/C-6.

daughters deserve nothing less. So why is it so hard for us as women to give ourselves the same tender loving care we give our children?

Whether or not you choose to have a hysterectomy is up to you and I respect that. But all of us owe it to ourselves and our families to make the most informed choices possible about what to do with our bodies. As the owners of some pretty complicated plumbing, we have the right to demand the best possible care by the best possible physicians using the best possible techniques.

Even the Fraser Institute says Canada has the sixth most expensive health insurance system in the OECD, yet we rank low for overall availability of, and access to, medical resources and the output of surgical procedures.[16] According to the institute, Canada ranks 13th (the US ranks 12th) out of 25 OECD countries on spending for hysterectomies per 100,000 population, spending almost twice what England, Ireland, Portugal, Hungary and Israel spend.[17]

So I ask you, are we getting value for our money if we have to wait a year or more for minimally invasive surgery when we need relief now?

Are we getting value for our money when Canadian women are spending between $25,000 and $100,000 of their own money to travel to the US for minimally invasive surgery when those same surgeries are available here?

Are we getting value for our money when some provinces are spending $30,000 to send women with advanced endometriosis to the US for surgery when we could keep the money here and put it towards upgrading physician training, buying state-of-the-

---

[16] Fraser Institute, *Value for Money from Health Insurance Systems in Canada and the OECD* (Vancouver: Fraser Institute, 2010), Introduction.
[17] Fraser Institute, *Value for Money from Health Insurance Systems in Canada and the OECD*, 8.

art equipment for the benefit of all Canadian women or creating centres of excellence in minimally invasive gynecology across the country?

Are we getting value for our money when the quality of and access to care a woman receives in Canada depends on where she lives?

These are difficult and complex questions with no easy answers. The hysterectomy epidemic stems from many things, which I will discuss in this book, not least of which is a cultural bias on the part of old-school gynecologists performing old-school surgeries.

If we can learn to stop smoking, wear seatbelts, use car seats, sleep our babies on their backs, not drink and drive, sneeze onto our sleeve, recycle and compost, we can stop offering hysterectomies as the default surgery for treating HMB in this country.

Now before you run to your computer to send me a message on Facebook saying how insulted you are that I would even suggest that hysterectomy is not always necessary for treating HMB, let me tell you I have heard from scores of women who say that hysterectomy was the best thing that ever happened to them, that it changed their lives for the better, that it ended their suffering and increased their enjoyment in life a hundredfold.

On the other hand, I have heard from women who say their lives have been ruined by the procedure. And some gynecologists have warned me that I may be raising false expectations in women by suggesting that these state-of-the-art alternative procedures are universally available when so few Canadian gynecologists are trained in these new procedures.

My answer to that is, "You have to see it to dream it." If you don't know Tim Horton's has a new kind of coffee, why would you ever go looking for it?

What I have discovered, through my own experience and while researching this book, is that there are at least 10 things you could be doing to get your bleeding under control that do not involve a hysterectomy. Some of these things can be done in the time it takes to make an appointment with your doctor. Others take longer, a lot longer.

In Canada, under our universal healthcare system, choosing to have a minimally invasive alternative hysterectomy, or an alternative procedure, is not for the faint of heart. It takes time to get a referral and even longer for surgery, not something you want to hear when you feel like you're bleeding to death. It is not a fast and easy fix. From the time I started bleeding heavily to the time I had my state-of-the-art procedures, almost two years had passed. For many women, it's more like five, six or even seven years.

A lot of people ask why I chose to prolong my suffering when I could have had a hysterectomy to solve the problem permanently, and much more quickly. To this day, I'm not quite sure I can articulate it. There was a lot at stake for me – my uterus, my womb, the place where I carried my children. It was just as much a part of me as testicles are for a man. All I can say is the woman in me said, "It just didn't feel right." The researcher in me said, "It wasn't medically necessary."

Show me the money

Please take what you read in the following pages and put it into this context: I am a patient, a researcher and a journalist. My experiences as a patient are my own; however, my findings as a researcher and a journalist are factual. You can trust that the information I have presented for this book is true, credible and based on extensive interviews with patients, gynecologists and other trustworthy sources. Although this book has been written by a Canadian about the Canadian healthcare system, most, if not all, of the medical and surgical alternatives to hysterectomy outlined in this book are available in most industrialized countries, *if you do your homework and go looking for them.* More importantly, my message of hope and empowerment is universal; and judging from the number of women who have contacted me from other countries, so is the level of suffering and frustration we all share. HMB is a problem worldwide so my hope is that women from around the world will benefit from the information I present.

Whether you live in Fredericton, New Brunswick, Philadelphia Pennsylvania, London, England or Christchurch, Australia, consider this book a starting place, a way to open a conversation about options with your doctor that you may not have had the courage or information to open before. I have interviewed some of the world's leading experts in minimally invasive gynecology, adolescent gynecology, oncology and genetics and have passed along their messages in language that we, as patients, can understand. Many of the physicians you will hear from are true visionaries, trailblazers if you will, who are charting a new course for the treatment of HMB by developing new treatment guidelines, new diagnostic and surgical protocols and most of all, new training courses for younger – and older – gynecologists who want to upgrade their skills. This new breed of gynecologist has our back and our front and I commend them for having the courage to speak out.

Finally, and perhaps most importantly, you will meet some amazing, courageous women who agreed to share their stories so that other women could benefit from their experiences. When I first began researching this book, I thought I was writing about Canadian women only. Now, as you will discover from reading this book and by visiting my websites (unhysterectomy.com and facebook.com/unhysterectomy), women from all over the world are contacting me with their stories. All of these women are just like you and me. They have suffered the ravages of heavy bleeding for far too many years and have chosen to cope in their own unique ways. Some did nothing, some chose hysterectomies and others chose every procedure in between, and I respect every one of them for the choices they made.

I must also say that many of these women are in their 20s and 30s, a fact that surprised me greatly. I thought I was writing a book for premenopausal women in their late 30s, 40s and early 50s, but after I created my Facebook page and my website I started hearing from much younger woman. Some of these women would have lost their ability to have children if they had not done their homework and shopped for a doctor who could help them without removing their uterus.

None of these women took their decision to seek treatment lightly, whether they chose a hysterectomy or not. It was something they wrestled with for years. Some of the stories you will read, including my own, may inspire or perhaps enrage you. Some of the comments from doctors may shock you. Some of the medical and surgical alternatives you will learn about will definitely challenge your thinking.

Too hot to handle?

This book may offend some women who think I am against hysterectomy. And yes, judging from the title you may very well get that impression. I will let you in on a little secret. I am not *against* hysterectomies. I am *for* making informed choices. I deliberately chose "The UNHysterectomy" to tick people off, to catch their attention, to enrage or inspire them enough to *start talking.* Sigmund Freud said the definition of insanity is doing the exact same thing over and over again expecting a different result. In other words, it's time to find a new solution to an old problem.

As women, we must awaken the sleeping giant within us to demand better for ourselves, for our daughters and for those who are working so tirelessly on our behalf. I am not naïve enough to think that one book can change the world. But we have to start somewhere, don't we?

My story:
How I avoided a hysterectomy

I knew as I lay in bed at two in the morning, soaking through a super-plus tampon and the two overnight pads I had taped together from front to back, that it would be another sleepless night. I dreaded getting out of bed to change my supplies. I had ruined enough underwear, nightgowns and sheets over the previous year to know that any sudden movement, even rolling over, could cause a major gush. Still, I braced myself, slowly squeezing my legs together as I rose to cross the bedroom floor. Damn, here it comes. Ploosh. Blood trickled down my thigh and onto the carpet as I fumbled my way in the dark towards the bathroom. Relief was on the way, at least for another two or three hours.

Bleeding profusely three days a month, losing sleep, keeping a change of clothes at work, not being able to concentrate because of my anemia and total exhaustion had become normal for me. As a single parent raising two adolescent girls and working two jobs, I was an absolute mess. Were it not for the love and support of my children, my family, my partner (now my husband) and my boss, I probably would have lost my job and my sanity. I needed help and I needed it fast.

Enough is enough, I thought as I trundled off to my family doctor for the third time in a year. "I can't take this bleeding anymore," I told her. "What's wrong with me?" Of course I was scared it was cancer. She listened attentively and could see I was in trouble. As a mitigating measure, she prescribed the blood-thickening medication tranexamic acid (brand name Cyklokapron), which I was to take every four hours during my heaviest days.

My doctor also sent me for a pelvic and transvaginal ultrasound. Both are used to diagnose irregularities so I was happy to at least be getting some kind of diagnosis. Many of us are used to pelvic ultrasounds, where the technician rubs jelly on your belly and waves a "magic wand" around to get a good picture of your insides. With a transvaginal ultrasound, the technician places a long transducer directly into your vagina. The probe is covered with a condom and a gel to make insertion and probing easier. The probe sends out sound waves, which reflect off your body's structures. The nearby computer receives the signals and uses them to produce a picture. The technician can then immediately see the picture on a monitor. I could see all kinds of things popping up on the screen but had no idea what it all meant until I got the results a few weeks later.

Diagnosis: Fibroids

My family doctor informed me that I had multiple fibroids growing inside the lining of my uterus, one as big as an orange, and growing bigger by the month. Fibroids? Never heard of them. In doctor lingo, I presented with the uterus of a three-month pregnancy. Some women present with a uterus as big as a five-, six- or even seven-month pregnancy.

Uterine fibroids, also known as leiomyomas, are non-cancerous tumours that develop on, or in, the lining of the uterus. It is estimated that up to 80 percent of women have fibroids, although only about 25 percent experience symptoms that can be diagnosed either through a pelvic exam or ultrasound.[18] Fibroids can cause severe bleeding, extreme pain or, for some lucky women, no symptoms at all. They are the leading reason for hysterectomies in North America, accounting for more hysterectomies than all gynecological cancers put together.[19] Fibroids can be as small as

---

[18] E.A. Stewart, *Uterine Fibroids. The Complete Guide* (Baltimore: John Hopkins University Press, 2007), 7.
[19] E.A. Stewart, *Uterine Fibroids. The Complete Guide*, 7.

a marble or weigh as much as 40 pounds and can be detected by ultrasound in almost 80 percent of all African-American women for reasons that are yet unknown.[20]

No one really knows what causes fibroids, except that estrogen (the female hormone our bodies produce during our childbearing years) makes them grow. Happily, fibroids usually stop increasing in size after menopause. A geneticist in Finland has found a gene that he believes may be linked to fibroids. I will explain this further in the Chapter 3.

Only three options?

My doctor referred me to a gynecologist whose office was a few minutes away from where I live. I remember it was a hot summer day when I arrived in his cool, air-conditioned office. Despite my excitement at finally getting help, I was having a particularly bad day. I don't take the heat well at the best of times, but with the heat and humidity, combined with a complete lack of energy and exhaustion from my anemia, I was a bit of a sitting duck. If that doctor had offered me a hysterectomy right then and there, I probably would have taken it, and I think he knew it, too. He could see the desperation on my face.

After a few short minutes, he appeared in the waiting room, calling my name, my chart in his hand. He was about my age, maybe a bit younger, and cheerful and full of enthusiasm. I suspected he had seen a lot of women in my position and knew how to handle us, or so I thought. We walked down to his office, or what I thought was his office. "Don't mind the mess," he said. "They're doing renovations on my office. I can assure you my surgical technique is a lot neater than this," he said, laughing.

---

[20] E.A. Stewart, *Uterine Fibroids. The Complete Guide*, 8.

Intuitive red flag number one.

I laughed along with him, nervously, scanning the piles of paper and office supplies strewn everywhere. After reviewing my chart, he explained I had three options: manage my symptoms until menopause, which doctors call watchful waiting; increase my dose of Cyklokapron; or have a partial hysterectomy to remove my uterus. "Your uterus lit up like a Christmas tree," he said, referring to my ultrasound, which I remember showed many coloured dots indicating where the fibroids were. He described my uterus as a "cancer nest" and said a hysterectomy was the only permanent way to solve my bleeding and remove any risk of developing uterine cancer down the road (even though I had no family history of uterine or any other cancer).

Intuitive red flag number two.

With language like that, I bought in. I was scared. I was so out of it and completely desperate to make the bleeding stop, I allowed him to pull me in. Still, I asked him what would happen if I did nothing for a while in hopes that things would get better on their own. He advised me that the fibroids would likely keep growing until I hit menopause, which was probably still several years away for me, and that without some sort of treatment my anemia would continue to worsen.

"How dangerous is anemia?" I asked him, thinking the mental and physical fatigue that was plaguing me were just (relatively) harmless side effects that affected my ability to function, but really nothing more sinister than that.

"If your body is losing that much blood, then your brain isn't getting enough oxygen to function," he said. "You could die of a heart attack. It's pretty serious stuff."

Intuitive red flag number three.

OK, now I was really scared. He told me my uterus was a cancer nest just waiting for the disease to strike, and then I find out I could die from a lack of oxygen to my brain. It was all too much for me to take in. I could feel a lump rising in my throat. "I'm pretty sure I'm going to have the hysterectomy, but I'd like to discuss it with my partner first," I said.

"No problem," he said. "Just give me a call and let me know what you decide."

I was devastated and confused. I remember walking out of there feeling like my world was about to come to an end. I was no stranger to surgery, having had a few minor procedures over the years, but this was different. This was a hysterectomy. It all seemed so big and overwhelming and beyond my ability to comprehend. Although I didn't know much about it at the time, I knew enough to be worried. Very worried. I phoned Gaston on my cell phone outside the doctor's office, crying. "I think I have to have a hysterectomy," I sobbed. "He said I could die if I keep bleeding this way and that it was probably best to take out my uterus so I don't develop cancer. I don't know what to do. I just want to stop bleeding."

Gaston talked me off the ledge and assured me that he would come with me to my next appointment. I actually went back twice more, first with my friend Lynne and then with Gaston. My mind was in such a complete fog I truly could not understand or retain anything the doctor was saying, so it felt good to have people I loved in the room with me.

I remember the day I said yes to the surgery. Gaston and I watched as the doctor practically leapt out of his chair, saying "I have the most admitting privileges of any gynecologist in Ottawa so I can get you in within the next six to eight weeks," he said, pointing to his wall calendar.

Intuitive red flag number four.

Although I found his enthusiasm completely inappropriate, I was hopeful because under the Canadian healthcare system you can wait more than a year for surgery, depending on how serious your condition is. So, after looking at the calendar more closely, I agreed and we booked the surgery. I just wanted the whole nightmare to be over. Gaston, however, slung one last salvo.

"Is there no other procedure than can help Holly without a hysterectomy?" he asked.

"There is a myomectomy, where we go in and cut out only the fibroids, but you don't want that. It's major surgery and even more bloody than a hysterectomy," he said. "We have to cut open the abdomen the same as we do with a hysterectomy, and there's no guarantee the fibroids won't grow back. Besides, I get paid more to do a hysterectomy," he said with a belly laugh.

Intuitive red flag number five.

Although many women rave about this particular doctor on RateMDs.com, other women complain profusely about his bedside manner, dismissive approach and outdated knowledge, a common complaint I hear from women across Canada about some of the gynecologists they are referred to.

So there I was, drained and exhausted, my brain in a fog, facing the prospect of major surgery. Although I was subconsciously carrying around those red flags, I was too scared, too shy or too desperate for relief to allow them to enter my consciousness. All I knew is that I was done.

I remember sitting on the couch one afternoon calling my sister Sue, who lived just outside Toronto, to tell her my news. She knew I was having problems and that I was leaning towards getting a hysterectomy. We often chatted about different programs she had seen on TV that talked about the after-effects of hysterectomy, some of which were not very pretty, such as bladder or bowel perforation and sexual dysfunction.

"You're going to have the surgery, Hol?" she exclaimed. "You're crazy!"

Intuitive red flag number six.

I remember it as if it were yesterday. Sisters have a way of sometimes speaking the truth without sounding judgemental. Anyway, knowing the fibroids were growing bigger by the day and the bleeding was getting worse, I ignored her, thinking it was my body and I could choose to do with it what I wanted.

If only

One warm and sunny September Saturday morning, three weeks before my surgery, Gaston was busy making pancakes and the rest of us were all doing our own thing. My daughters were 14 and 12.

The phone rang. I recognized the long-distance ring and almost didn't answer it, thinking it was a telemarketer. But it was my 86-year-old dad. He and Mom lived in Toronto, in the same house Sue and I and our older sister, Lesley, had grown up in since the 1950s.

"Holly," Dad said sternly. I didn't put much stock in his tone as Dad can be pretty gruff sometimes. Mom was in the throes of early dementia so he took over the task of calling us. "It's Susan. There's been an accident. We don't know much. Pete's on his way to the hospital and said he would phone us when he got there."

The girls wondered why my face had dropped. "It's OK, girls," I said. "Auntie Susie's been in some kind of accident and Uncle Pete's on his way to the hospital. It's probably just a broken leg or something."

Gaston and I ran upstairs to the bedroom to wait for the next call. I sat on the bed, waiting in agony.

Fifteen minutes later, the phone rang again.

"Dad, what happened?" I asked, my heart thumping out of my chest.

"It's your sister. She's..."

"No!" I screamed as I threw the phone to Gaston and collapsed on the bed. I burst into hysterical sobs; the girls came running upstairs and I told them what happened. All of a sudden, in a flash, at 9:30 on a Saturday morning, my beautiful, funny, soul mate sister was gone. Boom. Just like that. No warning, no chance to say goodbye or I love you. She was only 52. Sue was the funniest, kindest person I knew, a talented artist, dancer, comedian, stay-at-home-mom after 30 years in the banking industry, and everyone – I mean everyone – who knew her loved her. She had a magical way of making everyone feel happy and good about themselves. Sue had died in a car accident coming home from her 11-year-old son's hockey practice, five minutes from home. She had driven her own car that morning because she was late drying her hair. Her son had decided to go home with his dad at the last minute.

There were some 300 people at her funeral, many of whom were hockey families who'd come to pay their respects. I remember I was having a particularly bad period the week it happened so on top of dealing with that, plus the brain fog, anemia, exhaustion and shock, I was numb and completely out of it.

You'd think Sue's death and the stress of the funeral and reliving our childhood through the eulogy I gave would have motivated me to want the hysterectomy even more. After all, it brought the promise of relief, which would have helped me, I thought, cope with the loss of my dear sister and with life in general. But I actually felt the opposite way. I began to think that if Sue could wake up one morning, do something as innocent as watch her son play hockey and then not come home, then maybe something might happen to me during or after my surgery. My doubts and the rawness of my grief were enough to make me cancel my hysterectomy. Suddenly, I had turned the whole "freedom to choose" thing upside down.

A miracle cure?

After we got home from the funeral (and our parents' 60th wedding anniversary party, which we decided to go ahead with because Sue would have wanted it that way), I went to see my family doctor for what seemed like the millionth time. She could see the grief on my face and my sheer desperation for something – anything – that would alleviate the bleeding.

To my surprise, she suggested I try a birth control device called the Mirena. She explained that the Mirena is an IUD (intrauterine device) that was approved in Canada for contraception and for treating heavy periods, and she thought it might help. I was worried because I'd been fitted for some of those awful copper IUDs in the 1980s and they always came out. Plus, the idea of having a foreign object implanted in my uterus was somewhat distasteful to my middle-aged brain.

The Mirena, I learned, is a plastic, hormone-releasing IUD that slowly releases the synthetic hormone levonorgestrel into the uterus; it lasts for five years.[21] Levonorgestrel is similar to progesterone, a sex hormone produced naturally by the body. I agreed to try it as a way to stop my period and buy me some time. The Mirena has actually revolutionized the way abnormal uterine bleeding is treated in North America and has given millions of women relief from their monthly bloodbaths. Others, however, report side effects such as pain, bloating, weight gain and headaches, to name a few.

I was one of the lucky fibroid sufferers for whom the Mirena worked. But at about $300, the Mirena is expensive, and it wasn't covered by my health insurance plan (although birth control pills were covered; go figure). Anyway, from the day I had the Mirena fitted, my heavy bleeding stopped. Hallelujah! I did spot for an entire year and had to wear a pad 24/7 but the nuisance factor was nothing, and I mean nothing, compared with the nightmare I had been living, so it was a godsend. One thing you should know, however, is that there have been cases of the Mirena perforating the uterus,[22] so be sure to talk to your doctor about the pros and cons before getting one. Again, it's all about informed consent.

So, after getting fitted with the Mirena and with my bleeding under control, I was finally able to think straight for the first time in more than a year. With renewed vigour and determination to solve my problem permanently without invasive surgery, I decided to do what most women love to do: go shopping. Except in this case, I was shopping for a doctor who could help me without removing my reproductive organs.

---

[21] www.mirena.ca.

[22] Bayer Pharmaceuticals. "Association of MIRENA (Levonorgestrel-releasing Intrauterine System) with the potential risk of uterine perforation," Public Communication (June 15, 2010).

I shopped online, made cold calls, talked to friends, scanned books and articles, and finally found a gynecologist who specialized in alternatives to hysterectomy. He had just moved to Ottawa three weeks earlier and his waiting list was already filling up. Still, I cannot express the profound sense of relief I felt when his receptionist said he would see me. From what I can remember, I think I broke down and cried at my dining room table. Was it relief, hope or vindication? Finding this doctor was like having a miracle dropped in my lap (pun intended).

Dr. Sony Singh had just moved to Ottawa to begin teaching obstetrics and gynecology at the University of Ottawa and to open a new minimally invasive gynecology clinic at the Shirley E. Greenberg Women's Health Centre at the Ottawa Hospital. Dr. Singh is one of the leading experts in Canada and around the world on minimally invasive gynecology, a growing sub-speciality of the gynecological profession worldwide.

I remember being so excited to meet Dr. Singh. His staff said he could see me within four months. OK, I thought; I can handle that. The Mirena® had my bleeding under control, so what's another four months? Armed with this information, I went back to the first gynecologist I had been referred to. I thought he would be as enthused as I was to know that I would be able to solve my problem without undergoing a hysterectomy. Imagine my horror when he refused to refer me to Dr. Singh! All he said was "No." I was so shocked I didn't know what to say. At that moment, I truly felt as though he didn't give a hoot about me or my bleeding and that he was only trying to protect his surgical fees and his ego.

Feeling desperate again, I went back to my family doctor, again, and asked for the referral to Dr. Singh. She agreed, so off I went four months later. I remember our first meeting as if it were yesterday. Dr. Singh explained all the options available to me (including a hysterectomy and others I had never even heard of) and asked that I take them all into consideration before making my decision. I thought about it and agreed to try some of the newer procedures he offered me, which the other gynecologist had not even suggested.

Three months before the procedures I decided to have, I had injections of Lupron (leuprolide acetate, discussed in Chapter 11) to shrink the fibroids before surgery. Lupron is a synthetic hormone that significantly reduces your estrogen levels and puts you into temporary menopause.[23] As a result, the fibroids start to shrink, which makes it easier to remove them during surgery. One thing I was not expecting, however, is that Lupron can increase your symptoms during the first few weeks of treatment.[24]

In my case, I had two such episodes, each of which lasted for about two hours. The first time it happened, I had to leave my daughter's 15th birthday party to go to emergency because the blood just wouldn't stop. Every time I moved or stood up, it flowed out of me like a river. My dress looked like I'd been stabbed in the groin. The second time, I was having lunch with a friend. When I got up to go to the bathroom, in a matter of seconds I soaked through my jeans from my crotch down to my knees. I had to wrap my friend's sweater around my waist just to get back to the office. After discussing the episodes with Dr. Singh, I learned that as Lupron shrinks the fibroids, they begin dying off, which can cause shedding or clotting. Or, in my experience, Niagara Falls!

---

[23] www.lupron.com
[24] www.lupron.com

Two months later, almost a year to the day after my sister died, I had two of the most high-tech, state-of-the-art alternatives to hysterectomy available in the world: a hysteroscopic myomectomy[25] to cut out the largest of my fibroids and a hysteroscopic endometrial ablation[26] to burn the lining of my endometrium to stop or reduce my periods.

The surgery

Both procedures were done by inserting an eight-millimetre scope called a hysteroscope into my vagina, through my cervix and into the cavity of my uterus. A tiny camera on the end of the scope projected a live picture onto two plasma screens above the operating table to show Dr. Singh exactly where to attack the fibroids and burn the lining of my endometrium. The whole thing took about 90 minutes.

A few hours later, recovering from general anesthetic (which I chose; I could have had a spinal [epidural] or regional anesthetic and watched the whole thing unfold), I was up and around – no pain, no pain killers, no incisions, no stitches and all my reproductive organs intact. I plunked myself down in the passenger seat of my car when Gaston came to pick me up, his jaw dropping from shock over how well I was doing. I took 10 days off work, mostly to recover from the fatigue caused by the anesthetic.

Dr. Singh later told me, "I could have been in there all day there were so many fibroids," but he assured me he had removed the largest of them, so I was happy. Very happy.

---

[25] Grace Liu, Lynne Zolis, Rose Kung, Mary Melchior, Sukhbir Singh, E. Francis Cook. "The Laparoscopic Myomectomy: A Survey of Canadian Gynecologists," *Journal of Obstetrics and Gynecology Canada 32* (Feb. 2010), 139.

[26] Victoria General Hospital Mature Women's Centre, Hysterectomy Alternatives Program, Victoria, BC. http://www.vgh.mb.ca/mwc/halt_surgical_ablation.html.

Three years later

So here I am, three years after my surgery, and I still feel great. I have not had a period since, except for a few months in 2011 and another flooding episode in the spring of 2011. I had another ultrasound, which revealed that one of my fibroids had grown back (one of the risks of having a myomectomy, which I fully accepted) to about the size of a plum. I also had an endometrial biopsy to rule out cancer, which, thankfully, came back negative. Luckily, the bleeding has stopped except for a bit of spotting now and then but judging from my hot flashes I hope that menopause is around the corner. Forty-three years of bleeding is enough for me!

As you can see, I was more resolute, or stubborn, than a lot of women might have been. My choice to avoid a hysterectomy was a very painful and personal decision but one that I stand by 100 percent. One thing I learned from the experience is that life is too short and far too precious to waste time second-guessing yourself. I made my decision and I owned it.

What I also learned is that we, as women, have to stick together and support each other, no matter what we decide. I would never dream of judging another woman for deciding to have a hysterectomy, although it may seem that way from my story so far. There are enough things to feel bad about in life without making others feel bad for the choices they make. Only you know what is right for you and your body, and yes, with the help of your doctor and your family, you have all the tools you need to make the most informed choice possible. That the choice I made was right for me was never more apparent than on the day of my surgery and for me, that's what it's all about: making the most informed choice possible.

I remember lying on the operating room gurney chatting with the anesthesiologist while we waited for Dr. Singh to finish scrubbing up. She and I talked about whether or not it was a good thing to have a hysterectomy. I remember her saying that if it was her, she would have had the hysterectomy, without a doubt. "I'm done having kids," she said confidently. "So why not?"

Now that I think of it, the woman in me says, "Yup, I can totally relate." The journalist in me now knows there are many, many reasons to ask "Why?" instead of "Why not?"

PART II
ABOUT HEAVY MENSTRUAL BLEEDING

Chapter 1
Normal vs. Abnormal Menstrual Bleeding

The curse. Aunt Flo. Big red. Whatever you call it, bleeding is what we do as women. Although Pliny the Elder may have been just a tad severe in his dissertation on the evils of menstruation, our blood has been the stuff of legend since the dawn of time.

Before we can understand heavy, or abnormal, uterine bleeding, we have to understand normal uterine bleeding. Will you excuse me for a second while I adjust my sanitary belt? Are you old enough to remember those? I can remember sitting on the toilet fumbling with my pad when I should have been playing with Barbie, Skipper, Midge and Ken. Believe it or not, I still have my copy of "Very Personally Yours,"[27] the little handbook they gave us in grade five at Dublin Public Elementary School in Downsview (north Toronto) in 1968. The booklet shows a beautifully manicured hand holding a white embossed invitation, stars twinkling in the background, inviting us to some kind of secret puberty party where all would be revealed about becoming a woman. The book was given out as a companion to Walt Disney's short film "The Story of Menstruation"[28] (you must watch it on YouTube; it's fabulous), which he produced for the International Cello-Cotton Company, now Kimberley-Clark. The film was shown to more than 105 million schoolgirls in North

> **Menstruation**
>
> *A fatal poison corrupting and decomposing urine, depriving seeds of their fecundity, blasting garden flowers and grasses, causing fruits to fall from branches, dulling razors... [contact with] menstrual blood turns new wine sour, crops touched by it become barren.*
>
> – Pliny the Elder, Natural History, 77 AD

---

[27] Kimberly-Clark Corp., *Very Personally Yours* (Toronto: Kimberley-Clark of Canada Educational Department, 1961).
[28] Walt Disney Productions, *The Story of Menstruation* (International Cello-Cotton Company, 1946).

America from 1946 onwards. Although I have not been able to find a credible source for this piece of trivia, some online commentators believe "The Story of Menstruation" was the first film to use the word "vagina."

"It's no use pretending menstruation isn't something of a nuisance, and sometimes, downright uncomfortable," the booklet says.[29] "But a goodly share of that discomfort is in the mind. For modern doctors know that fretting can create sickness, even pain, when there's no physical cause for either. And thinking about menstruation as being 'unwell' – or dramatizing little irregularities – has made a part-time invalid of many a perfectly healthy girl." No wonder so many women of my generation just kept quiet about their symptoms. I guess they never knew about adolescent endometriosis back then.

Why women bleed

I realize it may seem ridiculous to explain the ins and outs of menstruation in this day and age, but you'd be surprised how many women don't really understand their periods or where they come from. I knew a woman once who was fairly overweight and had no idea she was pregnant until she went into labour! We have to understand how our bodies function in order to understand how something like a hysterectomy can affect us, for better or worse.

A recent study by the American Urogynecologic Society (AUG)[30] revealed some alarming research about women's misconceptions about the female reproductive system and the consequences of hysterectomy. Dr. Oz Harmanli and his research team surveyed 1,273 adult women in Springfield, Massachusetts,

---

[29] Kimberly-Clark Corp., *Very Personally Yours*, 9-10.
[30] Oz Harmanli, "Hysterectomy Misunderstood by Many U.S. Women," Press release (Washington: American Urogynecologic Society, Sept. 2011).

and Los Angeles, California. The women were questioned about hysterectomy and its perceived effects on sexual and reproductive function. Ninety-four percent of the participants were aged between 18 and 59 years; 48 percent were Latino, 38 percent Caucasian, and eight percent African-American and six percent were "others." The findings were startling to say the least:

- When asked the meaning of hysterectomy, 22 percent of women included removal of ovaries and Fallopian tubes in their definition. The precise meaning of hysterectomy is the removal of the uterus only, although removal of the ovaries and tubes may occasionally be necessary.

- 13 percent did not know the uterus was necessary to get pregnant.

- 44 percent did not know if a total hysterectomy eliminated cervical cancer. The cervix is the opening part of the uterus and a total hysterectomy includes removal of this part. It is not possible to develop new cervical cancer after a total hysterectomy.

- 41 percent thought they would continue to need pap smears after a total hysterectomy. A pap smear, a test for cervical cancer risk, is not needed after total hysterectomy, which includes removal of the cervix, unless the hysterectomy is performed because of cancer.

- 64 percent incorrectly thought they would start menopause by having their uterus removed. In fact, it is our ovaries that determine menstruation and menopause, whether they stop emitting hormones naturally or through surgical removal.

- 30 percent did not know whether removing the uterus would stop menstrual activity.

- 35 percent expected a change in sexual function after supracervical hysterectomy, which removes only the body of the uterus and preserves the cervix.

- 11 percent believed sex would be less enjoyable after hysterectomy, although according to the study there is "good quality" data confirming that hysterectomy does not affect sexual function in the majority of women.

"More comprehensive counseling is imperative for women who are younger, lack college education, and are on public assistance," said Dr. Harmanli in a news release from the AUG. "As physicians, we must raise the bar in women's health care and take steps to educate patients about the details and implications of all treatment options."

The female sexual organs

Although nature gave us everything we need to bear children, she also included some other parts just for fun. Understanding how these bits and pieces work together is very empowering, especially when you're deciding whether to keep some of them or not.

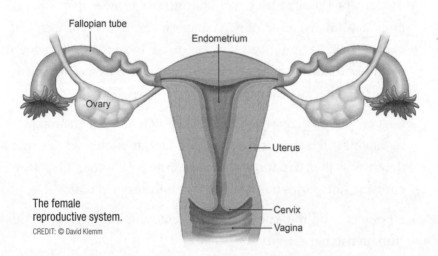

The female reproductive system.
CREDIT: © David Klemm

Labia majora

Labia majora literally means "large lips." The labia majora are the large folds of skin on the outside of your vagina that protect everything nearby, like your "pleasure centre," the clitoris. Each lip has two surfaces - an outer layer covered with pubic hair and a smooth inner layer containing glands that secrete oil and sweat.

Labia minora

The labia minora, the "small lips," are two small folds inside the labia majora, surrounding your vagina and urethral opening (the other hole, where your pee comes out). These protect the opening of your vagina.

Bartholin's glands

Bartholin's glands are two tiny glands just outside the opening of your vagina at five and seven o'clock. Their entire job is to secrete mucus to provide lubrication to make penetration easier. Unfortunately, these glands are a common site for pimple-like abscesses that may require surgery to relieve the pain and swelling.

Clitoris

Clitoris actually means "little hill." The clitoris is full of thousands of tiny nerve fibres whose sole purpose is to give us pleasure. Reach down and you can find your clitoris right below your pubic bone above the labia minora.

Vagina

The vagina is a muscular, elastic, tubular canal leading from the vulva (the labia, clitoris and vaginal opening) to the cervix of your uterus. Your vagina can vary in width and length and becomes thicker and longer during sex. Your G-spot is located at the front wall of the vagina.

Uterus

The uterus, your womb, is a pear-shaped organ deep in your pelvic cavity. It's divided into two parts, the cervix and the corpus. The opening in your cervix, which expands during childbirth to allow your little ones to be born, also allows sperm to enter and menstrual blood to leave (and leave and leave and leave). The corpus is an expandable, hollow area where, during pregnancy, the fertilized egg implants itself on the uterine wall and continues to grow inside the uterus.

Cervix

The cervix is the lower third of the uterus, forming the neck of the uterus and opening into the vagina.

Ovaries

Ovaries are wondrous glands, about the size and shape of almonds, that sit just above the Fallopian tubes on either side of the uterus. Each is responsible for producing hormones and eggs. Every month during ovulation (boy, do I remember *that* pain), either the right or the left ovary produces a mature egg, ready to be fertilized. Did you know that by the fifth month in the womb, you already have more eggs than you are ever going to need – some five million?[31] But by the time you get your first period, you have only about 400,000 left. Ovaries are an extremely important part of the female reproductive system so I urge you to read my chapter about ovary preservation. Our ovaries produce vital hormones that continue to protect our heart and lungs, even after menopause.[32]

---

[31] Lennart Nilsson and Lars Hamberger, *A Child Is Born* (New York: Delacorte Press, 1990), 17.
[32] Lynne Shuster, Brandon Grossardt, Bobbie S. Gostout and Walter A Rocca, "Prophylactic Bilateral Oophorectomy Jeopardizes Long-Term Health," *Menopausal Medicine* 18, no. 4 (Oct. 2010): S1-S5.

Fallopian tubes

The Fallopian tubes are just that – tubes that connect the ovaries to the uterus. Fully developed eggs produced by the ovaries travel to the Fallopian tubes, where they are fertilized by sperm. The fertilized egg, called a zygote, then moves to the uterus, where it implants itself in the uterine wall.

What triggers your first period?

Doctors call it menarche, or the start of menstruation. Menarche usually occurs about two years after we start growing breasts (one friend of mine jokes that she's still waiting for hers). Nowadays menarche can happen anywhere from age 11 to 14, although studies have shown that girls are getting their periods younger and younger these days.[33] Breast cancer researchers are particularly disturbed by this trend – they say that when puberty arrives earlier, exposure to estrogen lengthens and increases the chance of developing breast cancer later in life.[34]

Menarche is triggered by signals coming from the pituitary gland in the base of the brain. The pituitary produces growth hormones that allow us to grow and mature. As we get closer to menarche, the pituitary gland starts sending out new signals for our bodies to produce the female hormone estrogen, which then makes its way into our blood streams and ovaries. Just before your first period, and every month after that until menopause, estrogen levels rise, causing the lining of the uterus to thicken in preparation for pregnancy. At the same time, an egg starts to mature in one of your ovaries.

---

[33] Sandra Steingraber and Jeanne Rizzo, *The Falling Age of Puberty in US Girls: What We Know, What We Need to Know*, The Breast Cancer Fund, 2007. www.breastcancerfund.org.
[34] Sandra Steingraber and Jeanne Rizzo, *The Falling Age of Puberty in US Girls: What We Know, What We Need to Know*.

About halfway through the menstrual cycle, the follicle containing the egg ripens and releases the egg to the surface of the ovary, where it sits for about 24 hours waiting to be fertilized by a sperm in the Fallopian tube. If the egg is fertilized, it continues along the Fallopian tube and then attaches itself to the uterine wall. If the egg is not fertilized, it breaks apart and dies, hormone levels drop, the thickened lining of the uterus starts to shed and we start to bleed.

If only it were always that easy.

Normal menstrual cycles and bleeding

According to most of the sources I have consulted, normal menstrual cycles should last anywhere from 25 to 31 days.[35] Normal periods should last about five days. Many of these same sources say we should normally lose between two and eight tablespoons of blood every month.[36] That might be right for women with normal periods, but those of us who've experienced abnormal uterine bleeding know we lose a lot more than a few tablespoons every month. A lot more.

---

[35] HealthLinkBC, "Normal Menstrual Cycle," 2011, www.healthlinkbc.ca/kb/content/special/tn9930.html.
[36] Canadian Women's Health Network. "The Inside Story," 1997, www.cwhn.ca/resources/pub/Sweet_Secrets/inside.html.

Chapter 2
Heavy Menstrual Bleeding: Prevalence, Signs and Symptoms

Imagine wearing an adult diaper, a super-plus tampon and an overnight pad while chairing an executive board meeting. Imagine meeting your future husband's best friends for the first time and leaving a red stain on their expensive white chair when you stand up to leave. Imagine sleeping on an air mattress on your bedroom floor three nights each month to avoid leaking blood all over your mattress. Imagine being told your life could be in danger if you have one more period like the one you had the month before.

These are not fictitious accounts created for dramatic effect; they are true stories from women who spoke with me for this book. I defy anyone, man or woman, to endure this kind of humiliation and suffering for years on end only to be told by their doctors it's all in their head or just a natural part of aging. That's what happened to Susan from Prince Edward Island: "Three years ago, I complained of heavy menstrual bleeding to my family doctor. He passed it off as menopause, telling me that I was depressed because I had come to the end of my useful life. He prescribed anti-depressants and sent me on my way. Three years later I still have the same symptoms – extremely heavy periods, foggy brain, forgetfulness, irritability, inability to concentrate, utter and complete fatigue and the list goes on."

What amazes me most about the stories women have shared with me is that every one of them, without exception, thought their pain and bleeding was normal, something they "just had to put up with." Of all the women I have interviewed, Maureen is the one whose story seemed to touch me the most. We chatted in the back room of her office, tucked away from her staff so we could have some privacy. I listened with a lump in my throat as she

49

matter-of-factly recounted the years of suffering she endured and the way she arrived at her decision to manage her bleeding without any kind of intervention, surgical, medical or otherwise. "You do what you have to do," she told me.

I got so caught up listening to Maureen, I never did find out what caused her heavy bleeding, but in a way it doesn't matter. It's all behind her now. At 59, she's fully menopausal and having the time of her life. Some might say Maureen was crazy not to have demanded a hysterectomy, but after exploring all her options and listening to the advice of her doctor, Maureen chose to go it alone. Maureen's story is a textbook example of abnormal uterine bleeding:

> I remember starting to bleed very, very heavily when I was 45. I finished menopause when I was 52 so I guess you could say I bled pretty profusely for seven full years. I was diagnosed with hemorrhagic anemia because I bled so heavily. I always had very regular and predictable periods. They would always last seven to 10 days and with very predictable cycles. I could tell you exactly when I ovulated and when I would start menstruating. So when the heavy bleeding started, it wasn't that it just came at an odd time; it came at a predictable time. But the bleeding would be very, very red, like real blood, movie blood, and not typical menstrual flow. When my periods were normal, I would have a bit of heavy bleeding in the middle of my flow and then it would taper off. This never tapered off. I would just continue bleeding.

> During the really heavy times, when I was in my late 40s and [early] 50s, I would have to change my supplies every two or three hours. And that would be super-plus tampons plus pad and that would be for several days. When it got really scary for me was when I started bleeding for two weeks solid, to the point where I actually thought that I was hemorrhaging. I have a sit-down job so whenever I would stand up, I could actually feel the blood flooding out of me. I remember seeing a client one Saturday morning and when I stood up to shake his hand, all of a sudden I realized I should have changed my tampon and pad because the blood started running right down

my legs into my shoes. I reached my hand out to shake his hand, and I think he was wondering why I didn't accompany him to the door. But I just stood there frozen, not wanting to move.

Bleeding like that was something I was very, very conscious of so I did a lot of things just to get through the day at work. I changed my style of dress. I wore dark pants, heavy stockings, draping sweaters that went below my hips so I could cover myself if I had to. I always had an extra pair of underwear, stockings and shoes at work and lots and lots of product. I timed my appointments so I could get to the bathroom to change my supplies every two hours. I was always very wary of upholstered chairs for fear I would leak all over them. I preferred to sit in plastic chairs but I remember one day I leaked all over my chair and had to ask the girls to help me get it out of the way so I could get another one to keep on working. I have stained chairs. I have had my car professionally cleaned because I leaked blood through my coat and onto the upholstery of my vehicle, and I have even pulled out of traffic on bridges because I had to vomit I was so nauseous from the cramping.

I made my physician aware of the discomfort I was having and the investigation into a possible hysterectomy started. I had the vaginal ultrasounds and I kept track of the number of days I bled and so on. The information that was given to me was that hysterectomy was a very drastic measure for something that could be temporary. Nobody knew how long it was going to last.

I was always optimistic, thinking that it was going to get better. Of course it didn't. It got worse. It affected my work, my energy level; I was anemic and I was always pale like a ghost. I was scared, really scared. I asked for a D&C [dilation and curettage, the surgical removal of part of the lining of the uterus] but my doctor said no because I would just have to come back and get another one. So I just decided that I would not have any surgery whatsoever and just live with it.

You do what you have to do and hope every month that it will get better. Eventually, my doctor started to become very concerned about my blood levels and did encourage me to have a hysterectomy. She actually threatened me and said if I had one more period like the one I had the month before I would have to be hospitalized. But I remember around that time it started to gradually taper off and I went into menopause. No breakthrough bleeding, nothing. Absolutely nothing. It just stopped. What a real relief.

It's been wonderful. I think the first thing I did was run out and buy the sexiest pair of underwear I could find. It is so freeing to be able to be more relaxed with people, to not have to worry about leaking all the time, to wear feminine clothes, to wear white in the summertime or something that floats away from your body. I didn't think something like that would matter to me but it does. It's actually quite lovely to be able to do that. I feel sexier than I ever have in my entire life. I can undress and look at myself in the mirror and I look great. I can work out. I can swim or play squash or do whatever I want instead of worrying or being embarrassed or self-conscious about leaving stains everywhere. I am glad I didn't have the hysterectomy because I think I'm still producing enough female hormones to make me feel feminine and sexy.

If I had had this much energy when I was younger I would have had a lot more fun and been a lot more relaxed. As for my career, I think I could have lived up to my potential more, or maybe even been prime minister.

Isn't it incredible how much more Maureen thought she could have accomplished in life if she had not had to contend with such embarrassing and debilitating bleeding every month? Although I am tremendously happy about the way things turned out for Maureen, I find her statements very telling. How many of us are there right now not living up to our potential or not living the lives we want to because of a so-called natural, everyday condition that keeps us incapacitated?

As women, we tend to come into our own late in life anyway, once our children are grown and are more capable of fending for themselves. Usually by the time we hit our 40s or 50s we're ready for some serious "me time." But if that me time is consumed with managing monthly bloodbaths and feeling wrung out most of the time, the chances of us having the time or the energy to start travelling or writing or knitting or climbing Mount Everest are pretty slim.

How common is abnormal uterine bleeding?

Although the statistics vary slightly between Canada, the US and Europe, depending on which studies you read, roughly 30 percent of women suffer from HMB at some point in their lives.[37] That means about one of every three or four of us is going through the same kind of hell Maureen went through to some degree. Can you imagine what that is doing to our quality of life? Our mental, physical and emotional health? Our incomes? Our families? Our workplaces? Our communities?

In 2009, researchers at the Johns Hopkins Bloomberg School of Public Health in Baltimore, Maryland, studied the financial and quality-of-life burden of dysfunctional (abnormal) uterine bleeding (not the result of any one "organic" cause) from the perspective of women who chose surgery to manage their symptoms.[38] Researchers measured the annual costs of women's out-of-pocket expenses for tampons, pads and prescriptions; the value of time missed from paid work and home management activities; health as it related to being able to function; and the greatest amount of money that could be spent on surgery to alleviate symptoms (keep in mind this was a US study). Researchers questioned the women about:

- What they were spending, if anything, on medication

- The number of pads or tampons they used on their heaviest day

- How their daily activities were affected

---

[37] George Vilos, Guylaine Lefebvre and Gillian Graves, "Guidelines for the Management of Abnormal Uterine Bleeding," *Journal of Obstetrics and Gynecology* 106 (2001): 1.

[38] K. Frick, "Financial and Quality of Life Burden of Dysfunctional Uterine Bleeding among Women Agreeing to Obtain Surgical Treatment," *Women's Health Issues* 19, no. 1 (Jan-Feb 2009): 70-8.

- Whether or not they took time off work

- How much money they spent on supplies

- How much money they lost by taking time off, if any

- Whether or not pain, anxiety or depression, usual activities, self-care, mobility or blood staining were issues they had to deal with, in general

The findings are startling:

- 95 percent reported pain and cramping.

- 93 percent reported staining their clothes.

- 93 percent reported tiredness.

- 84 percent reported interference with their daily activities.

- 70 percent reported using 15 pads or tampons on their heaviest day.

- 47 percent reported missing one day or more from work per period.

- 25 percent reported being confined to bed at least one day per period.

But to my mind, the most startling finding of all is this: researchers found that the level of function in women in the study group was similar to that in patients:

- With visual impairment associated with age-related macular degeneration (loss of vision due to a damaged retina)

- Entering cardiac rehabilitation after suffering a heart attack or having bypass surgery to open blocked coronary arteries

- With malignant esophageal dysphagia (the feeling of food getting stuck in your throat)

This is incredible! This is the only piece of scientific literature I have been able to find that actually quantifies the debilitating symptoms of HMB in relation to other life-threatening conditions such as heart attack and blocked arteries. I have said it before and I'll say it again: abnormal uterine bleeding is not just a quality of life issue. It is a health issue worthy of the same examination, analysis and appropriate health policy as any other debilitating condition.

As for the cost of HMB, the average woman spent US$333 (in 2007) per year on tampons, pads and prescriptions, while money lost in paid work and home management amounted to $2,291 per patient per year. The study also found that women whose symptoms were treated surgically, at a cost of about US$40,000 either for hysterectomy or less-invasive surgery, and whose quality of life would improve as a result, could "earn back" about one-third of a year in "quality-adjusted life years" for every year they lived symptom-free until menopause. Imagine how much our lives would improve if we could have an extra 100 days or so, symptom-free, every year. Maybe we really could run for prime minister.

What this study proves to me is that women who suffer from abnormal uterine bleeding are missing out big-time. Considering we make up 50 percent of the Canadian workforce, that means *millions* of us are not operating at full capacity. And when we're not operating at full capacity, we're not living up to our potential. And when we're not living up to our potential, we're missing out on the opportunity to live our best lives and contribute to our families, our communities and our society in a much more meaningful way.

Varying definitions

Until recently, there was no term for abnormal uterine bleeding that everyone could agree on. Is it abnormal uterine bleeding, dysfunctional uterine bleeding or heavy menstrual bleeding? How much blood is too much? How should menstruation be measured and using what protocols? How can you define abnormal if some heavy bleeders never complain of their symptoms while some lighter bleeders might?

For the record, here are some of the more common terminologies and definitions used for abnormal uterine bleeding:

- **Abnormal** or **benign uterine bleeding** is defined as changes in frequency of menses, duration of flow or amount of blood loss.

- **Dysfunctional uterine bleeding** is abnormal uterine bleeding in the absence of disease, often the description used for changes in bleeding caused by variations in hormone levels with or without ovulation. This term is outdated and will be replaced by international guidelines with more practical descriptions.

- **Menorrhagia** is heavy menstrual bleeding occurring over several consecutive cycles during the reproductive years. It's defined as blood loss of more than 80 millilitres per cycle. Monthly blood loss in excess of 60 millilitres may result in iron deficiency anemia and may affect your quality of life.

- **Dysmenorrhea** refers to painful menstruation.

Newer, more practical terminology

As I mentioned, Canadian gynecologists recently introduced the term "heavy menstrual bleeding" to describe our condition and at the time of writing in early 2012, new gynecological guidelines were being developed for its treatment. (Please check my website, unhysterectomy.com, for updates.) The change is based on making the term as patient-centred as possible and making it more understandable. Heavy menstrual bleeding is defined as excessive menstrual blood loss that interferes with a woman's physical, social, emotional or material quality of life.

Symptoms of heavy menstrual bleeding

Whatever you call it, abnormal uterine bleeding can be diagnosed fairly easily if you have any of the following symptoms:

- Needing to change a tampon or pad more often than every two hours

- Needing to use a tampon and a pad together, or two tampons or two pads together

- Wearing adult diapers

- Flooding, or loss of control of menstrual flow, particularly upon standing

- Getting up at night to change your supplies

- Changing your work or social schedule to accommodate your heavier flow

- Bleeding or spotting between periods

- Periods less than 28 days apart or more than 35 days apart

- Time between periods changing each month

- Passing clots

- Bleeding for more days than normal or for more than seven days

- Bleeding past menopause. **If you are bleeding past menopause, put down this book and call your doctor immediately. It could be the sign of something very serious**

Without any sort of *universally* accepted definition of abnormal uterine bleeding, or consistent protocols for diagnosing and treating it, how can doctors or hospitals even begin to take the condition seriously? I remember the day my husband rushed me to the hospital when I had that Lupron – induced flooding episode while waiting for my surgery. There was blood everywhere. I almost fainted in the car on the way there and I was really scared. I walked into the waiting area and of course everyone looked at me like I'd been stabbed in the groin. My dress was soaked. After waiting for 10 hours to finally be seen, I remember how perplexed the doctor seemed when I asked him why I bled so much. I was used to blood after almost two years of living with fibroids, but this was like a river that just wouldn't stop. Every time I moved or walked it just poured out of me like water from a tap.

"Well, you've certainly lost a significant amount of blood," the doctor said. "But your blood work came back OK so I really don't know what's going on."

At that point, I probably knew more about HMB than he did. I now know I should have demanded that the hospital call my gynecologist. Imagine if there were no set guidelines for treating people with diabetes or heart conditions. Doctors would be just as perplexed in deciding what to do in emergency situations as the doctor who assessed me was.

I am heartened, however, that the Canadian Society of Minimally Invasive Gynecology (a fairly new organization started by a handful of forward-thinking gynecologists such as Dr. Singh and others you will meet later) is developing new guidelines for abnormal uterine bleeding for gynecologists across Canada. Once published, these guidelines will replace the old guidelines set by SOGC, which have not been updated since 2001. As well, some teaching hospitals have developed new, interactive, state-of-the-art modelling tools to help gynecology students learn step-by-step ways of diagnosing and treating abnormal uterine bleeding based on clinical evidence.

Chapter 3
Common Causes of Heavy Menstrual Bleeding

One of the challenges in establishing standards for the diagnosis, measurement and treatment of abnormal uterine bleeding is that no two women menstruate the same way. And perception plays a big role in determining how we view the heaviness of our flow. Unlike diabetes, cholesterol levels, blood pressure or something as common as a fever, which have longstanding diagnostic criteria, there are no exact, medically agreed-on, quantifiable standards for measuring how much is too much blood to lose during menstruation or between periods.

Scientists have found that the way we perceive our flow determines the way we describe it, which in turn affects how it is treated. In other words, the whole process is largely anecdotal. As far back as 1966, scientists compared how much women bled with how much they thought they bled. In one study, 11 percent of women who perceived their loss as light actually lost more than 80 millilitres of blood, while 27 percent of those who complained of a heavy flow actually measured in the lower part of the normal range.[39]

> There is no good classification system for the heaviness of periods. When I was a student, one of the senior doctors said that whenever he got a call from a patient complaining of heavy bleeding, he would ask whether the bleeding was so heavy that blood would fill up her shoes if she were standing without a pad. If she replied that it was, he would ask her to come in immediately. Although an exchange like this would be considered patronizing today, it does illustrate the difficulty of describing excessive bleeding.
>
> – Dr. Elizabeth Stewart,
>   author of *Uterine Fibroids.*
>   *The Complete Guide*

---

[39] I.S. Fraser, C. Pearse, R.P. Shearman, P.M. Elliott and R. Markham, "The Efficacy of Mefenamic Acid in Patients with a Complaint of Menorrhagia," *Obstetrics and Gynecology* 58 (1981): 543-51.

My cup runneth over

There is one way to measure your flow. One day while I was researching this chapter, I stumbled across a quirky little product called The Diva Cup. Basically, you put this cup inside your vagina over your cervix, *et voilà!* Apparently, it collects blood for up to 12 hours. I cannot imagine wearing one of these cups back when I was taping pads together every 90 minutes, but if you stick the cup in for even a few minutes to see how much blood flows into it, it could actually be quite a good little measuring tool.

What causes abnormal uterine bleeding?

Many things can influence the frequency of our periods and the amount of flow, such as hormones, stress, being overweight or underweight, exercising too much, certain medications and certain health conditions.

With the exception of certain conditions such as ovarian, uterine or cervical cancer, which can produce abnormal uterine bleeding even after menopause, most abnormal uterine bleeding can be attributed to other, more benign conditions, such as fibroids, adenomyosis (thickening of the uterus), endometriosis, polyps, cysts, polycystic ovary disease, uterine hyperplasia (when the lining of the uterus becomes too thick) and von Willebrand disease.

Treatments

The range of treatment options is pretty much the same for all of these conditions, as I will explain in Part IV. I suggest you brush up on the treatments before meeting with your doctor so you can work together to devise an appropriate treatment plan. Before we explore some of the causes of abnormal uterine bleeding, I want you to ask yourself two very important questions before you decide on any course of treatment (which will be discussed in greater detail later in the book):

- Do I want to have children?

- Do I want to prevent pregnancy?

Fibroids

Fibroids are nasty, non-cancerous (not even pre-cancerous) masses of muscle within the uterine wall that account for more hysterectomies in Canada[40] (and the US) than almost any other condition. These tumours can lie dormant and cause no symptoms at all or they can grow to the size of a watermelon. Some women with fibroids bleed for a few days while others continue past a week or 10 days. In 2008/09, 35 percent of hysterectomies in Canada were performed for the treatment of fibroids.[41]

The thing about fibroids is they creep up on you so slowly that you hardly know they're there until you start having symptoms. That's exactly what happened to Mercy, a lovely, confident young woman from Toronto who started having symptoms while she was going to university in London, Ontario: "My problems began in 2006, when I noticed something in my lower abdomen like a sort of mass that I could move around. It was strange. I thought it was gas or something at first. I was in university at the time and got caught up with school and studies and didn't think anything of it. I had always had painful and heavy periods but this was different. By the time I moved back to Toronto to do my post-grad, it was starting to hurt. It was more of a presence and I couldn't hide it under my clothes anymore. It was this huge bulge. I found out later my uterus was the size of a five-month pregnancy."

---

[40] Canadian Public Health Agency, *Health Indicators 2010*, 38.
[41] Canadian Public Health Agency, *Health Indicators 2010*, 38.

Like so many women I have spoken with, Mercy was bounced around from one doctor to another trying to get a proper diagnosis, a process that included going for cancer testing.

> They did an MRI and couldn't say conclusively that it wasn't cancer. I was like, "Oh my God." I was terrified. My doctor said she would have to do a hysterectomy because if it was cancer the cells could spread. At this point my mom was coming with me everywhere and I remember so clearly her saying, "Mercy, you just have to do it because it's too serious now. Why would you risk your life just for this?" referring to my uterus. I said, "Mom, I'm 26. I haven't even used this part of me, you know? Why should I give up all of that?"

> It was really emotional. I was crying but I just said no. The doctor tried to convince me to keep the surgery date because if I cancelled and changed my mind I would have to wait another six months. It was frightening because she said if I did have the surgery she would have to cut me vertically because of the size of the mass and not to be overly concerned about aesthetics because my health was more important.

> I had already invested a few hundred dollars in natural remedies from the UK that supposedly would shrink the fibroids so when I left the doctor's office I went directly to the local naturopath store and stocked up on some more things that would balance my hormones and do this and do that and cleanse. I remember doing that right after. My mom was with me and I was quite calm. I was just very firm in my decision somehow. I don't know how to describe it but it was grace-of-God type stuff.

I am happy to report that Mercy was eventually referred to Dr. Singh in Ottawa and underwent a myomectomy for the removal of her fibroids, which solved her bleeding while preserving her uterus. (See Chapter 16 for more on myomectomies and my website, unhysterectomy.com, for more on Mercy's story.)

Fast facts about fibroids

The four different types of fibroids are classified by where they grow:

- Just beneath the lining of the uterus (submucosal)

- In the middle of the uterine wall (intramural)

- Under the outer covering of the uterus (subserosal)

- Under the outer covering of the uterus on a stalk either inside or outside the uterus (pedunculated)

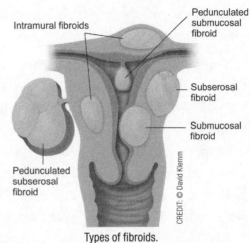

Types of fibroids.

Symptoms

- Heavy or prolonged periods

- Pelvic pain

- Pressure on your belly, bladder or back

Symptoms typically decrease after menopause.

Cause

No one really knows what causes fibroids except that the female hormones estrogen and progesterone make them grow. Once our bodies stop producing those hormones during menopause, the fibroids stop growing.

"There do appear to be abnormalities of the blood vessels in fibroids," says Dr. Elizabeth Stewart of the Mayo Clinic in Rochester, Minnesota. "And there are abnormalities of specific molecules that influence bleeding and blood vessel function. But exactly how you get from this lump of muscle to heavy menstrual bleeding isn't really known."

Dr. William Parker, co-author of *A Gynecologist's Second Opinion: The Questions and Answers You Need to Take Charge of Your Health* (Plume, 1996) and a clinical professor at the UCLA (University of California, Los Angeles) School of Medicine, often ponders the mystery of fibroids because of the havoc they wreak on women and the fact that they are the leading cause of hysterectomies in North America. "Fibroids have never made sense to me. Ten thousand years ago, why was the gene for fibroids even preserved? Why do women even get fibroids?"

In her chapter on the genetics of fibroids, Dr. Stewart explains that although there is no exact known cause of fibroids, we have to assume our genes might have something to do with them. "It is increasingly clear that the genes people are born with cause them to be at risk for certain diseases. The genes are really the instruction for all the body-building parts, and they can cause malfunctions. We begin life with instructions that program our body to respond in particular ways. Beginning with this assumption, we believe that genes influence a woman's ability to develop fibroids and also probably influence whether they cause bleeding, increase in size, or are quick to form again after surgery,"[42] says Dr. Stewart.

Since being diagnosed with fibroids in 2007, I have spent a lot of time thinking about them and wondering if they're hereditary. As the mother of two daughters, I want to know everything I can about these troublesome benign tumours. There are some rare fibroid syndromes that can be clustered with other disorders, such as, hereditary leiomyomatosis and renal cell carcinoma (HLRCC) syndrome. In families with HLRCC, men and women experience

---

[42] E.A. Stewart, *Uterine Fibroids. The Complete Guide* (Baltimore: John Hopkins University Press, 2007), 33.

fibroid-like lesions; these individuals are also at increased risk for developing a rare type of kidney cell cancer. However, it is imperative that we differentiate between these rare hereditary fibroid syndromes and the kinds of fibroids found in most women. Still, if fibroids are the leading reason for hysterectomy, and generations of women from the same family have had hysterectomies, there must be some correlation. While science is a long way from discovering the cause of fibroids, researchers at the University of Helsinki in Finland have discovered a mutation in the MED12 (mediator complex subunit 12) gene, an x-chromosome gene, which is altered in up to 70 percent of fibroids. Their discovery attracted worldwide attention when it was announced in 2011. The study's corresponding author, Dr. Lauri Aaltonen, cautions women from getting too excited too soon, especially where the issue of heredity is concerned.

"Our finding is not about heredity but rather a somatic mutation, or a mutation which occurs during life, regardless of any genetic predisposition. I want to be very clear about that. There is no indication so far, though there may be in the future, that the MED12 mutation may have anything to do with hereditary susceptibility."

MED12 is involved in the process that turns genes into proteins inside cells. It's an important distinction because genes tell proteins what to do. The finding may help explain the conversation going on between the MED12 gene and the MED12 protein, which could one day help explain the genetic makeup of fibroids and how they form.

But what does this all mean, really? Mireille Cloutier is a Canadian Certified Genetic Counsellor in Ottawa. "As in any negotiation, without a mediator, things can go awry. Mutations in a key area of the MED12 gene can disrupt the protein's function. In the case of fibroids, this seems to be causing changes in the way certain genes are expressed (turned on and turned off) in the smooth muscle of the uterus, somehow driving the formation of fibroids. How the altered MED12 protein contributes to the formation of tumours [doesn't appear to be known as yet]."

Still, although the road to finding causes and cures for disease is a slow process, built brick by brick with findings such as this, Dr. Aaltonen is clearly enthused about the discovery. "Finding this specific mutation area in most leiomyomas [fibroids] gives us an exceptionally good starting point to develop targeted medical treatments to curb the growth of these tumours. But this is something that we need to aim for in the long-term. Perhaps we'll never get there, but you understand my point. This is a goal, a distant goal towards which we need to work. Equally, I would hope that at some point we have drugs available which, for example, if they do not cure the lesions, they reduce their size or stop them growing, which would, in many cases, reduce the need for surgery. So I would be very optimistic in the very long run. This finding is a giant step towards understanding why fibroids arise, but towards design of targeted therapies it is an early step. Let's hope the journey has begun."

Adenomyosis

Adenomyosis, also a benign condition, occurs in about 10 percent of all women.[43] Like fibroids, very little is known about the condition.

---

[43] American Association of Gynecological Laparoscopists, "Abnormal Uterine Bleeding," 2012, www.aagl.org//.

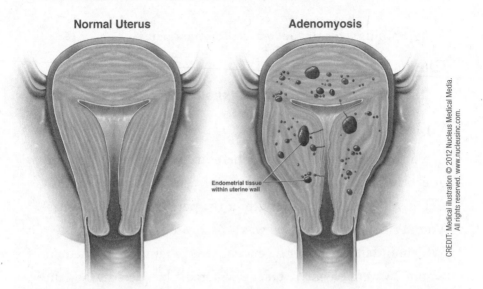

Normal Uterus   **Adenomyosis**

Endometrial tissue
within uterine wall

These images illustrate the difference between a normal uterus and a uterus with adenomyosis.

Fast facts about adenomyosis

- Tissue from the lining of the uterus (called the endometrium), which should be found *only* in the lining of the uterus, grows within the muscular walls of the uterus (the myometrium).

- The tissue can become irritated, form scar tissue or form fluid-filled cysts.

- Adenomyosis typically occurs in women in their late childbearing years (their 30s or 40s).

Symptoms

- Heavy, painful periods
- Bleeding between periods
- Passing blood clots during periods
- Tenderness in the lower abdomen
- Feeling of tenderness in the bladder or rectum

Symptoms typically decrease after menopause.

Cause

The cause of adenomyosis is unknown.

Von Willebrand disease

Von Willebrand disease is a hereditary bleeding disorder that affects approximately one to three percent of the population.[44,45] Ten percent of all women with heavy periods have the disease.[46] Von Willebrand disease was discovered by Dr. Erik von Willebrand in 1926 after he encountered a family of 66 people, of whom 23 were bleeders. Of the 16 female bleeders in the family, five died from bleeding, including a 13-year-old girl who died of uncontrollable bleeding during menstruation.[47]

Von Willebrand disease is really about clotting. People with the disease have blood that takes longer to clot. Normally, when people bleed, small blood cells called platelets go to the site of the bleeding and cause it to clot, thereby causing the bleeding to stop. People with von Willebrand disease are missing a protein in their blood called the von Willebrand factor, the protein which allows our blood to clot. Curiously, many people live symptom-free and may be unaware they even have the disease while others are diagnosed after a serious accident or surgery.[48,49]

[44] F. Rodeghiero, G. Castaman and E. Dini, "Epidemiological Investigation and Management of Women with Inherited Bleeding Disorders: Survey of Obstetricians and Gynecologists in the United Kingdom," *Hemophilia* 12 (2006): 405-12.

[45] E.J. Werner, E.H Broxon, E.L. Tucker, D.S. Giroux, "Prevalence of von Willebrand's Disease in Children: A Multiethnic Study," *Journal of Paediatrics* 123 (1993): 893-8.

[46] E.A. Stewart, *Uterine Fibroids. The Complete Guide*, 55.

[47] E.A. von Willebrand, "Hereditare pseudohaemophilic," *Finnska laekaellsk Handl* 68 (1926): 87-112.

[48] Canadian Hemophilia Society, "Von Willebrand disease," www.hemofilia.ca (accessed 2012). *An Introduction to von Willebrand disease.*

[49] Canadian Hemophilia Society, "Von Willebrand disease," www.hemofilia.ca (accessed 2012). *An Introduction to von Willebrand disease.*

Fast facts about von Willebrand disease

There are three types of von Willebrand disease.[50]

- **Type 1** – This is the most common type of von Willebrand disease, accounting for about 75 percent of all cases. People with type 1 are missing some von Willebrand factor. Some people have no symptoms while others have mild symptoms such as mild bruising, nasal or gum bleeding or bleeding longer than usual from cuts.

- **Type 2** – This is the second most common type of von Willebrand disease, accounting for about 25 percent of all cases. People with type 2 von Willebrand disease have enough von Willebrand factor; it just doesn't work properly.

- **Type 3** – This type of the disease is the most serious and is extremely rare with only about one in 500,000 people being affected. People with type 3 have very little von Willebrand factor and are at risk for more frequent bleeding, which if left untreated, can be dangerous.

According to the Canadian Hemophilia Society, von Willebrand disease often goes undiagnosed because "many doctors are not familiar with it." The society also says "many women with heavy, prolonged menstrual bleeding, who have not responded to hormone therapy, could be advised to have a hysterectomy."

Symptoms

Bleeding a lot is the main symptom of von Willebrand disease. The severity of the bleeding is different for each person. Symptoms of von Willebrand disease include:

- Excessive bleeding from the time of your first period
- Hemorrhage following childbirth
- Bleeding relating to surgery
- Bleeding associated with dental work

---

[50] Canadian Hemophilia Society, "Von Willebrand disease," www.hemofilia.ca (accessed 2012). *An Introduction to von Willebrand disease.*

If you experience two or more of the following symptoms, ask your doctor for testing:

- Bruising greater than five centimetres (2.5 inches) once or twice a month
- Nosebleeds once or twice a month
- Frequent gum bleeding
- Family history of blood disorders

Cause

Von Willebrand disease is usually passed down through families. It is the most common bleeding disorder present at birth (congenital), but most cases are mild. Men and women are equally likely to have von Willebrand disease.

Blood thinners and menstruation

I have not seen the issue of blood thinners and menstruation reported in any of the literature on abnormal uterine bleeding, beyond warning women with von Willebrand disease not to take blood thinners because of their blood's limited ability to form clots. The only reason I am even aware of the relationship between taking blood thinners and heavy menstrual flow is because of Sherri, who suffers from an autoimmune disease called antiphospholipid syndrome. Sherri experienced terrible bleeding episodes until she learned that taking blood thinners such as warfarin can substantially increase your flow.

Unlike von Willebrand disease, in which blood takes longer to clot, antiphospholipid syndrome, also called Hughes syndrome or sticky blood syndrome,[51] presents the opposite problem.

---

[51] T. Holden, *Positive Options for Antiphospholipid Syndrome* (Hunter House, 2003).

Antiphospholipid syndrome causes blood to clot more readily than normal.[52]

> When I first started taking warfarin no one told me, and the literature didn't tell me, about what warfarin does for your menstrual flow. It was crazy heavy, a real surprise based on flow and also colour. I mean, it was red, red, like theatrical makeup. It was like, "Oh my God. I'm dying." Honest to God, it was like CSI.
>
> Coincidentally, after being diagnosed, I got my period on the day I went to see my thrombosis doctor. I was literally leaking when I was talking to him but I didn't know I was leaking until after I left. So because I was scared, I went to the local hospital and they said, "Oh yes, you're on warfarin. Your periods are going to be heavy." I was really rattled the first time it happened because I didn't know how I was going to cope with the logistics of this. The flow was so heavy I had to pack myself with two overnight pads, like a submarine sandwich bun between my legs. I have an executive job in a male-dominated environment where I have to sit at meetings for long periods of time and I didn't want to have to be excusing myself every hour to change my supplies. I had already ruined a brand new pair of Gap jeans and a chair at work and I didn't want to have to go through that again.
>
> So I devised a system where I put super-plus pads inside a Depends so I could at least walk around or attend meetings. I had to watch what I wore so I didn't look like I was wearing a bustle. It was a really good system but Depends are really expensive. I remember one time driving to the US to find a deal on Depends and I had to ask my boyfriend to declare some of them for me because just buying four packages put me over the daily [customs] limit.

Fast facts about blood thinners and menstruation

People taking blood thinners, or anticoagulants, tend to bleed and bruise more easily than normal. As we know from experience, such tremendous blood loss can lead to anemia.[53]

---

[52] T. Holden, *Positive Options for Antiphospholipid Syndrome*.
[53] T. Holden, *Positive Options for Antiphospholipid Syndrome*, 119.

Symptoms

- Very heavy menstrual bleeding (at least twice the normal amount)

Endometrial polyps

Most of us know someone who has been diagnosed with polyps, or perhaps have had them ourselves. Polyps are also benign masses that can overgrow inside your uterus, causing mild pain and heavy periods. Unlike fibroids or adenomyosis, endometrial polyps start growing in the lining of the uterus (the endometrium) and stay there.

Fast facts about endometrial polyps

- Endometrial polyps can be long, like fingers, or rounded, meaning they can sometimes be confused with fibroids.[54]

- Polyps can cause irregular or heavy bleeding, but not the kind of long, heavy bleeding associated with fibroids or adenomyosis.

- Endometrial polyps can range in size from a few millimetres to several centimetres.

- Women at an increased risk of developing polyps are obese, have hypertension, have had polyps previously or are taking the medication tamoxifen for the treatment of breast cancer.[55]

Symptoms

Signs and symptoms are the same as with any abnormal bleeding:

- Prolonged or heavy periods

---

[54] E.A. Stewart, *Uterine Fibroids. The Complete Guide*, 157.
[55] Victoria Hospital Mature Women's Centre. Hysterectomy Alternatives Program. "Common Diseases of the Uterus," www.vgh.mb.ca (accessed 2012).

- Bleeding between periods or after intercourse

- Bleeding or spotting after menopause

- Menstrual-like cramps (endometrial polyps seldom cause pain)

Cause

The exact cause of endometrial polyps remains unknown but they seem to be influenced by circulating hormones.

Ovarian cysts

Ovarian cysts can be normal because every month tiny sacs full of fluid that contain an egg get ready to mature. They form on the surface of the ovary and then disappear after the egg is released. There's a difference between ovarian cysts, which are usually harmless and symptomless, and ovarian growths, which can be caused by other problems such as cancer. Most ovarian cysts go away without treatment.

Important to know

Some growths can be tumours, whether malignant or benign, and may need to be removed to test them for cancer. Ultrasound is very useful in helping guide treatment.

Symptoms

- Pain or aching in your lower abdomen, usually mid-cycle

- A delay in the start of your period

- Bleeding between periods

Some ovarian cysts can twist or rupture and bleed. Symptoms include:

- Sudden or severe pain, often with nausea and vomiting

- Pain during or after intercourse

Cause

If a mature egg is not released, or the sac closes, it can swell up with fluid, forming what is called a functional ovarian cyst.[56]

New guidelines are afoot

Before moving on to one of the most devastating and painful conditions of all – endometriosis – I want to assure you that there are movements afoot within the Canadian gynecological community to address the inconsistencies in the way these conditions are diagnosed and treated. New guidelines are being developed by SOGC. The previous guidelines had not been updated since 2001. As soon as the guidelines are released, I will post a link on my website, unhysterectomy.com, so you can read them, think about them and take them to your doctor so you can have an informed discussion about forming a treatment plan.

---

[56] Alberta Health. "Functional Ovarian Cysts," 2012, www.myhealth.alberta.ca.

Chapter 4
Endometriosis: A Special Case

Endometriosis is a common and sometimes debilitating condition experienced by women of reproductive age. This disease causes pelvic pain and is sometimes associated with infertility.

Endometriosis is the growth of tissue, similar to the kind that lines a woman's uterus, elsewhere in her body. That "elsewhere" is usually in the abdomen. This misplaced tissue responds to the menstrual cycle in the same way that the tissue lining the uterus does: each month the tissue builds up, breaks down and sheds.

Menstrual blood from the uterus flows out of the body through the vagina; however, the blood and tissue from endometriosis has no way of leaving the body. This results in inflammation and sometimes scarring (adhesions), both of which can cause the painful symptoms of endometriosis and may contribute to difficulty getting pregnant.

Even though endometriosis has been researched extensively, it is a complex disease that can be challenging to diagnose and treat. Many

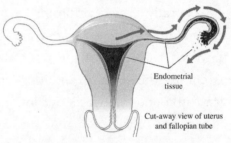

Endometrial tissue

Cut-away view of uterus and fallopian tube

This view of the anatomy of the uterus and Fallopian tube reveals one way in which the membranous mucous tissue from the lining of the womb may enter the pelvic cavity causing endometriosis.

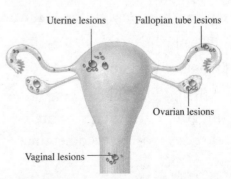

Uterine lesions   Fallopian tube lesions

Ovarian lesions

Vaginal lesions

Various lesions caused by endometriosis.

symptoms of endometriosis – severe, painful menstrual cramps; painful intercourse; and gastrointestinal upsets such as diarrhea, constipation and nausea – are similar to those for a wide variety of other conditions. As well, each woman with endometriosis will experience symptoms differently, depending on the location and extent of her endometriosis. This means that the combination of treatment options that work for one woman may not necessarily work for another. That's why it may take years for a woman and her healthcare professional to identify the extent of her endometriosis and find an effective treatment.

Symptoms[57]

Generally, the symptoms experienced depend on where the endometriosis is located and how extensive the growth is; however, there is not always a direct correlation between the extent of the disease and the symptoms. Some women have very little endometriosis but lots of pain and others have severe endometriosis with no pain.

In fact, some women with endometriosis may not experience any symptoms at all, and will never be aware they have the disease. But for other women, the pain associated with endometriosis can lead to fatigue, feelings of depression and isolation, problems with sex and relationships, and difficulty fulfilling work and social commitments.

Common symptoms[58]

The most common symptom of endometriosis is pelvic pain. This pain often occurs before or during menstruation, but may also be experienced at other times.

---

[57] Society of Obstetricians and Gynecologists of Canada, www.endometriosisinfo.ca. Reprinted with permission.
[58] Society of Obstetricians and Gynecologists of Canada. Reprinted with permission.

- **Severe menstrual cramps**. Menstrual cramps caused by endometriosis are different from normal menstrual cramps – they are more severe and may begin earlier in the menstrual cycle and last longer.

- **Painful intercourse**. Endometriosis can cause pain deep in the abdomen or pelvis during or following sex.

- **Painful urination or bowel movements**. With endometriosis, this type of pain may be experienced during menstruation. In cases where the bowel and bladder are severely affected by endometriosis, pain may be felt even between periods.

- **Lower back or abdominal pain as well as chronic pelvic pain**. Some women may experience abdominal and pelvic pain that is not associated with their menstrual cycles, but which occurs on a daily basis and which has lasted for six months or longer.

- **Other gastrointestinal upsets such as diarrhea, constipation and nausea**. For women with endometriosis, these symptoms may be experienced during menstruation.

Rare symptoms[59]

In very rare cases, the growth of endometriosis is very extensive and the following symptoms might be experienced, usually when you are having your period.

- **Leg pain or sciatica**. This type of pain suggests that the endometriosis is affecting nerves.

- **Rectal bleeding or blood in the urine**. This type of bleeding suggests that the endometriosis is affecting the bowel or bladder.

---

[59] Society of Obstetricians and Gynecologists of Canada. Reprinted with permission.

- **Shortness of breath**. This symptom suggests that the endometriosis may be affecting the lungs or diaphragm.

Endometriosis facts and statistics

- Approximately 176 million women and girls worldwide suffer from endometriosis, 8.5 million in North America alone.

- The average woman is 27 when she is first diagnosed with endometriosis.

- Endometriosis is one of the top three causes of female infertility. While it is one of the most treatable, it remains the least treated.

- Abdominal and bowel symptoms linked to endometriosis are commonly misdiagnosed as irritable bowel syndrome.

- Endometriosis is often misdiagnosed as pelvic congestion or pelvic inflammatory disease.

- Many infertile women with endometriosis experienced debilitating painful periods as teenagers but were misdiagnosed.

- Many women suffer silently because they feel that their pain, especially pain associated with sexual intercourse, is just too personal to discuss with their gynecologist. This is more common in some cultures than others.

- Many cases of endometriosis can be successfully treated with laparoscopic excision surgery. Hysterectomy should only ever be considered as a last resort.

How serious a condition is endometriosis?[60]

When I set out to write this book, I struggled with whether or not to include information about endometriosis beyond the basic facts. That may sound peculiar, given that the disease is perhaps the most crippling of all benign conditions associated with pelvic pain and abnormal uterine bleeding. The reason I hesitated is that my book deals with bleeding caused by benign conditions such as fibroids, polyps and cysts. Although endometriosis is still classified as a *benign* condition, there is a growing school of thought within the medical community that endometriosis is not a benign disease.[61]

Dr. Linda Griffith, professor of molecular thermodynamics and Director of the Massachusetts Institute of Technology (MIT) Center for Gynepathology Research, suggested in her November 2011 address to the 40th Global Congress of the American Association of Gynecological Laparoscopists (AAGL) that *non-malignant* is a better word than *benign*. Patient advocate Lone Hummelshoj was quick to praise Dr. Griffith for her position by including it in her news roundup on endometriosis.org.

> *I can't tell you the number of bright, intelligent, well-educated women I have seen who have had to suffer with various types of debilitating symptoms for years before being able to find an appropriate intervention. Endometriosis is a perfect example. On average, women suffer for seven years and go through a number of physicians before they actually reach a diagnosis and begin appropriate interventions. There's something wrong with that.*
>
> – Dr. Nicholas Leyland, President, Canadian Society of Minimally Invasive Gynecology; Professor and Chair, Department of Obstetrics and Gynecology, McMaster University

---

[60] Society of Obstetricians and Gynecologists of Canada, www.endometriosisinfo.ca. Home page, 2012. Reprinted with permission.

[61] Linda Griffith, "Endometriosis Is Not a Benign Disease," Address to the 40th Global Congress of the American Association of Gynecological Laparoscopists, Nov. 2011.

Please bookmark endometriosis.org if you're looking for an authoritative resource on endometriosis. Hummelshoj is the Chief Executive of the World Endometriosis Research Foundation, Secretary General of the World Endometriosis Society and publisher/editor-in-chief, endometriosis.org. She is a powerhouse of knowledge on endometriosis and certainly an inspiration to me, as a fairly new patient advocate.

"The word *benign* is used in the medical community in references to diseases that are not cancerous. From the patient/scientist perspective, however, Professor Griffith urged that any form of symptomatic endometriosis be referred to as *non-malignant* in order to capture the significant morbidity this disease exerts on the daily lives of patients.

"The use of the term *non-malignant* also highlights that certain pathological processes are shared by endometriosis and various forms of cancer, and that the respective research communities might learn from each other! The surgical community, in fact, has been extraordinarily receptive to building closer ties to the basic science and engineering communities, as shown at the AAGL by featuring a scientist as a keynote speaker!"

In other words, women with endometriosis are hanging on every word from the gynecology community these days for any sign of a cure or new treatment. Melissa, a 39-year-old mother of two in Toronto, has just been diagnosed with endometriosis after 10 years of pain and heavy periods. "My mother has it, my sister has it, my aunt has and now I have it. The doctor has just told me I have a lesion on my liver, so I am anxious to see what he comes up with for a treatment plan."

Katrina from Winnipeg has the double misfortune of having both adenomyosis and endometriosis, which unfortunately can go hand in hand. Katrina has decided to go ahead with a hysterectomy because she simply can't take it anymore.

The women in my maternal line, as far back as we can trace, have had a predisposition to endometriosis. I recently had a spell of bleeding that lasted 51 days and could only be managed by taking progesterone. The bleeding and clots were enough to seriously upset and disconcert me and my child (who mistakenly walked in on me in the bathroom during this time period).

I am always tired. I seldom have the energy to do anything more than the basic things around my house. I was on iron supplements until the bleeding was controlled and will probably continue with them, in a far lower dose, now.

I understand that hysterectomy is invasive surgery and not to be undertaken lightly. But I honestly can say I do not wish to risk the resumption of bleeding on that scale.

I've suffered my whole life with cramps during my cycle, which began when I was seven and then stopped for a year when I was 12. After that, it became horrific. I want the hysterectomy. I want to know it's gone and over and that I won't have to deal with these problems again.

Sadly, Dr. Singh sees patients like Katrina every day. Here is a special message from Dr. Singh for women suffering from endometriosis to let them know they are not alone and that there is help available.

Endometriosis is a disease that women carry silently. A woman who has endometriosis and is suffering in pain or has infertility from this condition will not show any external signs. My patients often tell me how they suffer quietly and when they do have significant pain that impacts work or school, others cannot and do not understand what they are going through.

The most significant aspect of this disease is to recognize that it is under- and misdiagnosed. Often women will not receive the proper diagnosis and hence treatment for up to seven to 10 years after they first present to the medical system. Also, traditional diagnostic techniques will often come up normal and will further delay diagnosis. Even ultrasound cannot see endometriosis until it is advanced. In fact, the economic burden of this disease is estimated to be $1.8 billion per year, most of which is the lost productivity of our young women in the workforce.

There are severe and debilitating outcomes from advanced endometriosis. It is like a cancer. It can spread anywhere in the body and invade other organs. It has been found everywhere, including on the ovaries and Fallopian tubes, on the bladder and bowel and appendix. However, it can invade into organs such as the bladder and bowel as well, which can result in significant symptoms and long-term damage. Endometriosis has also been found in the brain (presenting as seizures at the same time as the period) or lung (which collapses with a period!).

Expertise in this area is limited. Initial stages of endometriosis can and should be managed medically, starting with the birth control pill and then moving on to other medicines as needed. Advanced cases require a whole team approach, which is virtually non-existent in Canada. There are a few surgeons who specialize in this field but they are overwhelmed with volume, and there is very little financial support for this condition.

When surgery is needed women must do their homework. Almost all cases can be managed through minimally invasive surgical techniques and fertility-sparing procedures that can be done and should be the priority in young women. Removing the uterus and ovaries is seen as the definitive solution; however, it is not necessary most of the time and should not be the standard of care in young women.

Through education, support and guidance, women with this condition can see a significant improvement in their quality of life. Physicians, nurses and health professionals must help empower women to search for the best care possible and that means providing all women with access to excellence in gynecological services.

A reason for hope

Two promising developments occurred in 2011 that should give Canadian women with endometriosis hope for the future. SOGC has developed new guidelines for the medical and surgical diagnosis, management and treatment of endometriosis.[62] I strongly recommend you download these guidelines by going to endometriosisinfo.ca. Even though they were written for the medical community, they are easy to understand. I also recommend that you print the guidelines and take them to your next visit with your gynecologist or family doctor. These guidelines are a breath of fresh air.

Pay close attention to the clinical tip to doctors on page 17 of the guidelines regarding surgery: "The decision to move to surgery in women with pain and suspected endometriosis should be based on clinical evaluation, imaging and effectiveness of medical treatment." The words "effectiveness of medical treatment," of course, could be open to interpretation, which is why it is even more important that you know your stuff when discussing your options. What is effective for one woman may be different from what works for another and could be influenced by a number of factors, including severity of symptoms, desired outcome (preserving fertility, relieving pain) and personal choice (absolutely wanting a hysterectomy or not).

The guidelines include a special section on endometriosis and adolescents, which I believe is required reading for every parent of a daughter who complains of excessive cramps and HMB.

Another promising development is that Health Canada has approved a new drug called dienogest (Visanne) to treat the pelvic

---

[62] Society of Obstetricians and Gynecologists of Canada. "Endometriosis: Diagnosis and Management," www.sogc.org/guidelines/documents/gui244CPG1007E.pdf (July 2010), S31.

pain associated with endometriosis. Visanne is designed to be taken orally and contains a powerful synthetic form of the female hormone progesterone called progestin. Although there is no restriction to duration of use, clinical studies evaluating Visanne for pelvic pain associated with endometriosis have not tested efficacy beyond 15 months.[63]

Our bodies produce progesterone naturally, primarily in our ovaries, and we secrete the hormone throughout our menstrual cycle and during pregnancy. It's what triggers our bodies to ovulate and menstruate.

Progestins, which are often prescribed on their own or in birth control pills, prevent the lining of the uterus (endometrium) from overgrowing, which in turn helps prevent ovulation and can prevent abnormal uterine bleeding. Progestins also help regulate periods for women and teens who do not ovulate regularly. Visanne contains a novel progestin called dienogest, which suppresses the effects of estradiol (the most powerful sex hormone we produce) on endometrial tissue and effectively reduces pelvic pain.

Taking progestin-only pills continuously, such as dienogest, will cause changes in menstrual bleeding patterns. Dienogest may also cause spotting, irregular bleeding or periods may stop altogether. Menstrual bleeding patterns become less regular after taking initial doses of dienogest but the frequency and intensity of bleeding tends to decrease with continued use. You should consult your physician if your periods become longer or heavier.

"Visanne is an important management option for patients with the disease, as it is proven to relieve the chronic, debilitating pelvic

---

[63] Correspondence with Bayer, Inc.

pain caused by endometriosis including menstrual pain and pain during sexual intercourse," says Dr. Singh. This is the first new treatment in more than a decade to help these women, which is encouraging."

Health Canada approved Visanne in November 2011; however, you should talk to your doctor to see if the medication is right for you.[64]

---

[64] Health Canada, "Notice of Decision for Visanne," www.hc-sc.gc.ca/dhp-mps/prodpharma/sbd-smd/drug-med/ nd_ad_2011_visanne_132174-eng.php. Nov. 2011.

Chapter 5
When to Seek Treatment

The decision to seek treatment for abnormal uterine bleeding is often difficult for women. We're supposed to bleed, right? It's normal to have cramps, correct? So who are we to say how much is too much? If you have even the slightest urge to let your inner mouse say, "What if my doctor thinks I'm a whiner?" then you need to set a mousetrap. Get yourself to your doctor's office now because the longer you wait, the worse your symptoms will become, and the longer it will take for you to see a specialist, whether you want a hysterectomy or not. And believe you me, if you think your suffering is bad now, try bleeding for a year while you wait to see a gynecologist.

Let me repeat this as well: **if you're bleeding past menopause, you *really* need to call your doctor. Bleeding after menopause *is not normal* and can be a sign of a serious problem. Call your doctor *today*.**

One of my theories about why some doctors diminish our symptoms is that they can't measure them. They're scientists; in their world, it's about what they see. In my world, it's about how I feel. How do you measure a heavy period? How do you measure pain? How do you measure "my life is in the toilet?" Until science develops internationally recognized, quantifiable tests for measuring pelvic pain and abnormal uterine bleeding, all that doctors have to go on is what we tell them. Even diagnostic imaging techniques such as ultrasound and MRI (magnetic resonance imaging) measure growths, not symptoms.

I've developed a tool called **The Flow Chart** (download a printable copy at unhysterectomy.com) to help you measure the frequency, length and volume of your periods; the pain you experience; and the toll all of it takes on your quality of life. You can download it from my website at unhysterectomy.com, fill it in and take it to your doctor. It will give your doctor an instant snapshot of your condition and something more to go on than "my periods are killing me."

FLOW

DESCRIBE YOUR FLOW

How many days
is your period?
_____

How often do you
get your period?
_____

Is it predictable or does
it come when it wants to?
_____

Do you bleed between
periods?
_____

Do you bleed after sex?
_____

Are you bleeding during
menopause?*
_____

VOLUME

Number of pads used per day
_____

Number of tampons used per day
_____

Number of pads and tampons
used at the same time
_____

Number of adults diapers
used per day
_____

Do you wear adult diapers at night?
  With or without pads?
  Tampons?
_____

Number of adults diapers
used per period
_____

How often do you change
your supplies?
_____

How often do you change your
supplies overnight?
_____

Do you soak through your clothes? _____

Do you soak through your bed linens? _____

Do you pass clots? _____

What size are they and how many
do you pass in a day? _____

PAIN

Level (1 to 10 – 1 being no pain,
10 being killer pain) _____

Where is your pain located? _____

How many over-the-counter
pain killers do you take per day? _____

How many prescription
pain killers do you take per day? _____

MEDICAL HISTORY

Do you have a personal or family
history of a blood disorder or HMB? _____

Do you have a history of
anemia or taking iron supplements? _____

Do you have a history of a
thyroid disorder? _____

Do you bleed during dental work? _____

Did you have any
postpartum bleeding? _____

Have you had heavy periods
since puberty? _____

Do you have a history
of easy bruising? _____

QUALITY OF LIFE

PHYSICAL

How would you describe
your energy level?
(Less than average, fair, average,
better than average)

_____

How would you describe
your ability to perform routine
tasks, e.g., housework, laundry,
groceries, childcare?

_____

Are there any disruptions
in your daily activities,
e.g., exercising, playing with
the children, going out?

_____

How would you describe
the quality of your sleep?
(Less than average, fair, average,
better than average)

_____

MENTAL

Do you have difficulty
concentrating?

_____

Do you have difficulty
understanding things?

_____

Do you have difficulty
remembering things?

_____

EMOTIONAL

Are you anxious?

_____

Are you depressed?

_____

Are you sad?

_____

SEXUAL

Are you interested in sex? _____

Are you enjoying sex? _____

Is sex painful? _____

Is your pain and bleeding
having an effect on your
intimate relationship? _____

PROFESSIONAL

How many days of work
do you miss per month? _____

How would you describe
your performance at work?
(Less than average, fair, average,
better than average) _____

FINANCIAL

How much money do you spend
per month on supplies? _____

How many days a month
do you lose from work? _____

How much money do you
lose in wages? _____

How much money do you spend
per month dry cleaning or replacing
soiled clothing or linens? _____

* Bleeding after menopause could be a sign of a serious medical condition. See your physician immediately if this is the case.

For a downloadable version of The Flow Chart, visit unhysterectomy.com. Fill it in and take it to your next appointment with your family doctor or gynecologist.

What to say to your doctor

Back in the day, going to the doctor was like going to the principal's office. If he said "jump," we said "how high?" Times are different now. Going to the doctor today is about conversation, not dictation.

"Women need to know that they're not subservient to their doctor anymore and that they need to have their questions and concerns addressed," says Dr. Jennifer Ashton, author of *Your Body Beautiful. Clockstopping Secrets to Staying Healthy, Strong, and Sexy in Your 30s, 40s, and Beyond.*[65] She is also the co-host of the ABC show The Revolution, also seen on City TV here in Canada. I first saw Dr. Ashton on *The Dr. Oz Show* on February 25, 2010, when she talked about various alternatives to hysterectomy.

"In the past, women were kind of put on autopilot by their doctors. If you weren't having a baby or a hot flash, you were in no man's land. Now, it's the antithesis of that. Women of that age are now at their most vibrant and most healthy and part of that includes knowing how to talk to your doctor if you're having problems."

Marion Grobb Finkelstein certainly agrees with that. Marion (MarionSpeaks.com) is a communications catalyst based in Ottawa and the Niagara Region who specializes in helping people communicate to connect. She has 30 years' experience in business and government so she is highly capable of teaching us something about talking to our doctors more assertively:

> There's an old saying that we have one mouth and two ears for a reason: talking and listening. Good communication is really two-way and listening is a big part of that. The other part is the responsibility we have as women to

---

[65] J. Ashton, *Your Body Beautiful. Clockstopping Secrets to Staying Healthy, Strong, and Sexy in Your 30s, 40s, and Beyond* (Penguin, 2012).

define what our message is, who needs to hear it and why, and to deliver it in a way that will serve both the sender and the receiver. That certainly plays out in terms of how we talk to our doctors. We are responsible for our own bodies and our own health, and nobody can advocate for us like we can.

Women of our era were brought up to respect certain professions and not to question things. Certainly our parents never did. My mother was a career, lifelong nurse from the war years in the Ottawa Valley, to nursing in St. Catharine's, Ontario, in the 60s, 70s and 80s. Eventually she became a director of nursing so she worked with doctors day in and day out and although she never questioned or challenged them blatantly, she did get her message across. I learned many things at her hand and one of the things was respecting the medical profession. With regard to communicating our message, it's important to realize doctors are in their position because they come with many, many years' experience and lots of training. They come to us offering a fantastic service. So I think the most productive thing for us to do is to start looking at our relationship with our doctors as a team. They are on our team and we want them in our court.

So how does that translate into us asking our doctor to take our symptoms seriously? "Before we engage our mouths, it serves us best to engage our brains," says Marion. "One way that we can do that is to prepare. Fill in your Flow Chart. Do your homework, research what might be causing your pain and heavy bleeding. When you walk into that office you want to be as prepared for the conversation as you would be for a presentation at work. The bottom line is we need our doctors. We need them to advocate for us because they know the system. They have what we need. So the way to present it is to acknowledge and validate their perspective so that you can work together to find a solution. The conversation might look like this: 'I know how busy you are and I know you don't have much time so I am here to ask if you could send me for an ultrasound and some blood work to determine why I am bleeding so much every month.'"

Ask a direct question, get a direct answer. Being direct and to the point saves everyone time and frustration. My family doctor works incredibly hard; I can see it in her eyes. I can see how overwhelmed she is. She has three children at home and a demanding practice so the more direct I am in communicating the reason for my visit and making specific requests, the faster the appointment will move for both of us.

Another very important area to consider before you see your doctor is what subconscious attitudes you might be bringing to the table. Dr. Christiane Northrup, author of *The Wisdom of Menopause*, calls this our "hysterectomy legacy."[66] As women, we learn a lot from what we hear as young girls around the house, in the yard, down the street and at weddings and funerals and we internalize those messages and file them away where they start to form our beliefs, without us even realizing it. Did your mother have a hysterectomy? Your grandmother? Your sister? Women in your community? Were their experiences positive or negative? We can be strongly influenced today by something we heard 40 years ago and not even consciously register it. And that, girls, is what leads many of us to choose a hysterectomy.

"There are historical, geographical and cultural differences in the way certain procedures have been done in the past and I expect it will continue in the future," says Dr. Ashton. "For example, in the United States, the Southeast has a massive hysterectomy rate, whereas in the Northeast, where I am in the suburbs of New York City, hysterectomy rates are much, much lower. Rates also vary due to ethnic background as well. I used to take care of a tremendous number of women, almost exclusively Hispanic women, and they

---

[66] C. Northrup, *The Wisdom of Menopause* (New York: Bantam, 2001), 262-3.

would come to their doctor at the age of 50 or thereabouts and almost make up a reason to want to have a hysterectomy."

Dr. Wolfman of the menopause unit at Mount Sinai Hospital in Toronto has seen those disparities first-hand. "I lived and practised in the US for seven years in the 1980s. At that time there were whole towns where it was difficult to find women with a uterus. That attitude is certainly different amongst my patients in downtown Toronto in 2012. Many with very severe symptoms will try every medical therapy in order to save their uterus."

> It's more of a personality issue than where you are in your career. I know a number of older gynecologists who are almost ready to retire, and probably would have, save for their stock portfolio at the moment, who are active in learning these new skills. I mean, it's their personality that they want to keep up, - they want to try new things. There are also people of my generation who are perfectly happy to do what they're doing and show no inclination to improve their skills either. So I think it's more of a personality issue.
>
> – 30-year-old gynecologist at a major Canadian teaching hospital

How we think and feel about our private parts is so personal, so much more complex and biased, if you will, than how we feel about any other body part, except perhaps our breasts. Our feelings about hysterectomy are as entrenched in us as women as they are in many of our doctors. Many Boomer gynecologists I have spoken with who are still practising in Canada and the US say they were never taught to avoid hysterectomies. They were taught that when a woman presented with painful and heavy periods the best course of treatment was to do a hysterectomy.

"Our profession is entrenched in terms of doing hysterectomies," Dr. Ernst Bartsich, a gynecological surgeon at Weill-Cornell Medical Center in New York, told CNN Health.[67] "I'm not proud

---

[67] Curt Pesmen, "5 Operations You Don't Want to Get – and What to Do Instead," 2011, CNN Health, www.articles.cnn.com.

of that. It may be an acceptable procedure, but it isn't necessary in so many cases."

Thankfully, many of those gynecologists have upgraded their thinking as well as their skills, or are starting to, and now offer women a much wider range of choices, not just hysterectomy. But I want you to be aware that women and doctors bring a lot of biases to the operating table that were formed long before you set your feet in those stirrups. Acknowledging, and perhaps challenging, your own bias, and that of your doctor, is an important step on the road to making an informed decision about how to treat your symptoms.

Here's another interesting bias many women have. How can we challenge the person who helped us bring our children into the world? Who coached us through morning sickness and who put our babies in our arms for the first time?

"It's a very wonderful bond," says Dr. William Parker. "That's what attracted me to doing ob-gyn. There's nothing like it in medicine. It's all fun and wonderful and so you have that bond. Then when a doctor who's doing mostly obstetrics and doesn't know how to do minimally invasive surgery says, 'Well, a hysterectomy is the right thing for you,' or 'There's nobody here who can do this laparoscopically,' or 'your fibroids are too big or you have too many,' women trust that person. I understand it but I think the day has come, through the Internet, that a lot of women are getting more information to make a more informed choice.

"Now they realize there are all these other alternatives and they're saying, 'Why didn't my doctor tell me that?' Every day in my office somebody says to me, 'Why didn't my doctor tell me this?' I used to be a little more protective of doctors. But now I'm a little less protective and I usually say, 'Because they don't know how to do it and they're not going to offer you something they don't know how to do.'"

So challenging our biases and doing our homework are two very important steps on the road to making an informed decision about how to treat your symptoms. In summary, Marion Grobb Finkelstein has created **10 tips** to help you make the most of your appointments with your doctors.

Marion and Holly's 10 Tips for Connecting with Your Doctor

1. **Take a friend or family member to your appointments.** If you're exhausted or anemic from losing too much blood every month, chances are your brain will be in a bit of a fog. Ask a friend or family member to come with you to your appointment to help you advocate for yourself. Write down your questions before you go and have your friend write down the answers so you can review them later. This type of note taking will help you keep track of who said what to whom.

2. **Respect your doctor's time.** Doctors are very busy people with many patients to see. Your first appointment may be only five or 10 minutes. Make every minute count by describing your symptoms as succinctly as possible.

3. **Respect your doctor's expertise.** Even though there are some exceptions (as there are in every profession), most doctors want the best possible outcome for their patients. Go into the appointment knowing you have a highly trained, highly knowledgeable expert in front of you. Don't assume the worst.

4. **Be polite but assertive.** You can catch more flies with honey than with vinegar. When seeing your family doctor, remember, he or she is the intermediary between you and the gynecologist

who will treat your symptoms. You need your family doc and want to maintain your relationship, so keep that in mind and let it guide your behaviour.

5. **Listen as much as you talk**. You're there to work together to find solutions. Listening is a big part of the equation. Tune yourself to "receive" mode when your doctor is talking.

6. **Be specific**. Explain why you're there and what you want. Don't just ask the doctor to "make it stop." Try something more like, "I'd like to discuss what my options are, from minimally invasive to maximally invasive." Throwing in a bit of doctor lingo never hurts!

7. **Show your doctor your Flow Chart**. It will give your doctor an instant snapshot of your symptoms.

8. **Be insistent**. Do not leave the doctor's office without a requisition for either blood work or a diagnostic test such as an ultrasound. If your doctor refuses to send you for tests, suggesting instead that you monitor your bleeding for a few more cycles, politely explain that you have been monitoring your symptoms and you would like to move on to the next step.

9. **Ask for a specific referral**. Remember, this is all leading up to getting the right referral to the right doctor for the right treatment at the right time. Ask your doctor if he or she knows any gynecologists in the area who specialize in less-invasive treatments for heavy periods. If your doctor doesn't, try finding one on your own and go back to your family doc for a referral to that gynecologist.

10. **Don't be afraid to fire your doctor**. If you're not getting what you need from either your family doctor or from the first gynecologist you see, and if other doctors in your area are

accepting new patients, leave your doctor. (Caution: don't "fire" your doctor until you have a new one in place). Call or write to explain why you're leaving the practice and to ask that your medical records be transferred to your new doctor. It won't likely come to this because most doctors want the best possible outcome for their patients.

In other words, be prepared and show some chutzpah!

PART III
ABOUT HYSTERECTOMY

Chapter 6
Types of Hysterectomy

The term "hysterectomy" dates back to Ancient Greece, when philosophy, science and medicine were intertwined. The word *hystera* means uterus or womb in Ancient Greek. According to some experts, the word is rooted in Sanskrit, which defines it as the upper part of a woman's reproductive system. The suffix *-ectomy* comes from the Ancient Greek word meaning "to cut out."

"In his Timaeus dialogue Plato does say that a woman's womb moves about her body [the 'wandering womb'] and characterizes it as a living being within her. The idea is found in Hippocrates, too," says Amber J. Porter, a PhD student in Greek and Roman Studies at the University of Calgary. "The womb's movements are thought to cause a number of different symptoms in the woman, including suffocation [called 'uterine suffocation'] and the woman is said to be 'hysterical.' It was an idea that stayed with medicine for a long, long time and has basically been used to explain all sorts of women's 'issues,' especially emotional ones."

Canadian writer and broadcaster Bill Casselman provides this explanation on his website, billcasselman.com[68]: "Ancient Greeks and more modern men too had the sexist notion that nervous afflictions were peculiar to women and were symptoms of various uterine maladies. Plato imagined that the uterus...was a separate spirit and animal part of a woman that only wanted to become pregnant. If it did not, this imaginary uterus-spirit wandered in a fit of mopish pique through the female body causing trouble.

---

[68] Bill Casselman, "The Word of the Day: Hysteria," 2012,
www.billcasselman.com/dictionary_of_medical_derivations/fifteen_hysteria.htm.

When it arrived at the brain, this hystera (womb animal) went totally postal and induced feminine hysterics."

Porter suggests we read the article by Helen King, an expert in Ancient Greek gynecological medicine, in the book *Hysteria Beyond Freud.*[69]

Today, hysterectomy is a confusing term. Technically, hysterectomy refers to the removal of only the uterus, yet the term is used by most of us to describe taking out everything that could potentially be removed, including the uterus, cervix, Fallopian tubes and ovaries. But there are more specific variations of the term to explain the differences in procedures that remove different parts. The more you know, the better equipped you'll be to discuss the options.

There are four types of surgery to remove our reproductive organs – three types of hysterectomy and what is known as a "salpingo-oophorectomy," or ovary and Fallopian tube removal. These procedures can be prescribed for the treatment of endometrial, ovarian or cervical cancer, or of any of the conditions I discussed in Chapters 3 and 4.

- **Complete, or total, hysterectomy.** The name is misleading because with this type of hysterectomy, only your uterus and cervix are removed. Your ovaries and Fallopian tubes are left behind. This is the most common type of hysterectomy.

- **Partial, subtotal or supracervical hysterectomy.** This type of surgery removes only the upper part of your uterus and leaves your cervix and other organs in place.

---

[69] Sander L. Gilman, Helen King, Roy Porter, G.S. Rousseau and Elaine Showalter, *Hysteria Beyond Freud* (Berkeley: University of California Press, 1993).

- **Radical hysterectomy.** This type of hysterectomy removes everything – your uterus, the upper part of your vagina, supporting tissues and usually your pelvic lymph nodes. This type of hysterectomy is usually performed to treat cervical cancer.

- **Salpingo-oophorectomy** is the removal of one or both of your Fallopian tubes and ovaries.

Methods

There are three ways to do a hysterectomy:

- Vaginal

- Laparoscopic

- Abdominal

SOGC has specific guidelines recommending vaginal hysterectomies as the best method by which to perform a hysterectomy, followed by laparoscopic hysterectomies and then abdominal. As previously stated, despite these guidelines, more than half of all hysterectomies in Canada continue to be performed abdominally.

Abdominal hysterectomy

Abdominal hysterectomy is the most common type of surgery. It is also the most invasive because it involves a large incision in the abdominal wall. Your doctor may also call this a "laparotomy." It can be done either through a horizontal "bikini" incision (called a "pfannenstiel" incision) or vertically (a "midline" incision) from just below the navel down to the pubic bone. The operation requires a hospital stay of three to five days and recovery takes about six weeks.

Incision   Uterus

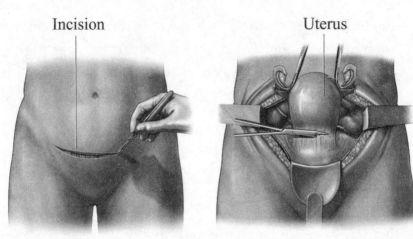

The two steps of an abdominal hysterectomy procedure as seen from the front. The first pictures a surgeon's hand cutting with a scalpel across the female abdomen. The second illustration displays a large laparotomy exposure with surgical instruments cutting along the lower border of the uterus.

My friend Delia had a radical abdominal hysterectomy a few years ago after suffering for years with endometriosis. We recently reconnected after losing touch for several years. When we got together, I learned that she had just had a hysterectomy a few weeks before. Although she was still off work and recovering from her surgery, not to mention dealing with going into menopause overnight, she appeared relieved that her suffering was finally over. Who can argue with that? "I was done," she said.

Before her hysterectomy, as with many women who suffer with endometriosis, Delia soldiered on, working full-time and raising two children with her equally hard-working husband. Meanwhile, the disease was worming its way into her bladder, her bowels and even her ureter (the tube that carries urine from the kidneys to the bladder). She says the pain was excruciating.

I was diagnosed with endometriosis the year before our second child was born in 1994. I had doubled over in pain at the office and later discovered a cyst on my ovary had burst. When they removed the golf-ball sized cyst

106

with laparoscopic surgery, they found endometriosis; they cleaned it up with a laser; and instructed us to try to conceive as soon as possible.

All was well for about 10 years when my GP discovered a grapefruit-size cyst. This time, the cyst and an ovary came out and we all hoped that I could wait another 10 years and natural menopause would put an end to the endometriosis before I needed surgery again. No such luck. Within two years, I was experiencing excruciating pain, which I managed with medication. When I think back, I recall feeling pressure on my bladder, too. But I didn't put two and two together and deduce the pressure might be something big sitting on my bladder.

Two years later, I became very sick with an infected cyst. I don't recall all the details. I do remember a raging temperature and that there was something very wrong with my belly. I knew it was endometriosis. I remember the specialist coming to talk with us after I'd had an ultrasound in the emergency department. And I'd already made up my mind. I'd already discussed it with my husband. The doctor was describing the options but my response was quick: Take it out.

I'd already had three abdominal surgeries in my life, all of which required months of recovery. I wasn't planning any more kids. I wanted to put an end to the surgeries and pain.

This time the surgery was hugely complicated by the infection. What was supposed to last two hours stretched into five. It required two blood transfusions and several specialists around the operating room table. One, I understand, was there to extract the endometriosis from my ureter. Two infectious disease specialists were involved. Afterward, my doctor held up her hands in the shape of a mango to show me how big the thing they removed had been.

I was relieved when it was all over. The only thing is that post-op I was having pain with intercourse. The specialist initially thought it was the result of the pain and carrying around the mango-sized cyst and that my body was compensating by tightening the muscles too much. I followed up with physiotherapy to learn how to relax the muscles [the opposite of Kegal exercises where you contract and release the muscles that support the pelvic floor]. But we eventually figured out it was just one of those everyday symptoms of menopause: the thinning of the walls of the vagina. Since then I use an estrogen cream that has taken 95 percent of the pain away. The cream was a miracle cure. It virtually restored our sex life within a week.

Early menopause was *nothing* compared to endometriosis. Hot flashes, I can deal with. Sex is different. But it's still very good. The orgasms are no less intense.

These are the stories that make pondering hysterectomy so complex. But perhaps there is nothing to ponder at all. Perhaps all we have is individual women making individual choices. My friend made the right decision and I am very, very happy for her.

Vaginal hysterectomy

A vaginal hysterectomy is less invasive than an abdominal hysterectomy because it involves no deep cuts through your belly. The operation is performed through an incision at the top of your vagina. First the uterus is pulled down into the vagina, and then the ligaments, cervix and blood vessels that connect the uterus to the rest of your body are cut and stitched. Vaginal hysterectomies are performed in hospital, under general or spinal (epidural) anesthetic. The operation requires a hospital stay of one or two days and a recovery time of about two to four weeks. Complication rates with vaginal hysterectomy are the lowest.

Another friend, Louise, loves to chat about her hysterectomy. She had a vaginal hysterectomy and has never looked back. It was a glorious, liberating end to 20 years of pure hell.

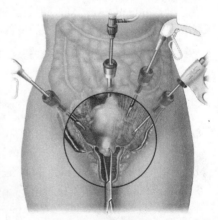

A vaginal hysterectomy scope orientation.

I was 12 when I first got my period and it got worse and worse every month. For me, I had the periods from hell and oh my, I suffered. It was a family thing because my mom had a hysterectomy and so did my sister. We all suffered.

My periods were heavy, like seven days long heavy. It was horrifying. I didn't go out to play. I didn't do anything because I had severe, severe cramps and blood clots. I'd wake up sometimes in the middle of the night and it looked like I had just slaughtered a pig in my bed. It was just full of blood. I'd get up and cry because it was 3:00 o'clock in the morning and I had to change the sheets and get up the next morning to go to school.

It got worse and worse the older I got, but I did get some relief after having my kids. But trying to work full-time [Louise is in the military] and raise two kids on my own while having these terrible, terrible periods was just a nightmare. It got so bad that I had chronic, chronic lower back pain. I'd wake up in the middle of the night and could barely even roll over because it was so painful. It was just crippling. I couldn't exercise. I had to take time off work. And forget about sex. Sex had always been painful for me but as I got older it became even more painful. It was excruciating.

It got to the point where I woke up one morning and instead of standing up on my two feet and walking to the bathroom, I actually crawled on my hands and knees to the bathroom because standing up was so bad. That's when I got dressed and I went to work and went down to the hospital and demanded a hysterectomy. I was so done.

Laparoscopic hysterectomy

Laparoscopic hysterectomy is minimally invasive because it, too, involves no major incisions. Laparoscopic hysterectomies are becoming increasingly available in Canada as more and more surgeons are trained to do them. For this procedure, the surgeon makes four tiny incisions in your belly, each about the size of a keyhole, and passes instruments and a laparoscope (a miniature camera attached to a slender telescope) down through the holes. Whatever the camera sees the surgeon sees on a video screen.

The uterus is then detached by laparoscopic instruments and removed through a small incision at the top of the vagina or through one of the small incisions in the belly if the surgeon is leaving the cervix in place. Using an instrument called a morcellator, the uterus can be cut into small pieces and removed through the tiny incision. Because the procedure is minimally invasive, recovery time is shorter than with open abdominal procedures. The hospital stay may be less than one day and you should be able to resume your normal activities after about one or two weeks.

Another friend of mine, Sue, recently underwent a partial hysterectomy to relieve the excruciating pain and heavy periods she was experiencing as a result of adenomyosis, which is often confused with fibroids. She often showed me how swollen her belly was and said she felt seven months pregnant all the time. I could see how anemic she was from losing so much blood every month and my heart went out to her. As the mother of two young children, and working full-time, she needed help. We talked several times about the choices I had made and about whether minimally invasive surgery was something worth considering.

After having an ultrasound and receiving the diagnosis, Sue was offered the full range of treatment options by her gynecologist, all the way from watchful waiting to hysterectomy. After weighing all her options, which included waiting eight months to see a surgeon who could perform minimally invasive surgery, she chose to have a hysterectomy. I applaud her for making the decision that was right for her and her family.

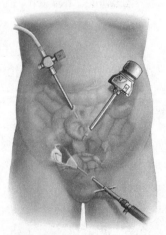

A laparoscopic hysterectomy scope orientation.

Sue was able to have the procedure done laparoscopically, and her surgeon removed only her uterus, leaving everything else intact.

"For me the laparoscopic vaginally assisted hysterectomy I had seemed worse than the necessary C-section I had with my second baby," Sue says. "Perhaps it was because I had to focus on the baby and get sleep when I could that I don't recall having so many problems. At least with the hysterectomy I could sleep during the day, which was really needed as I was so tired. My children were at daycare or at school so I could focus on myself. I took five weeks off work and returned to work for part days for three days before trying full-time.

"I thought I would be ready to return to work after two weeks but soon realized that I needed more time to rest and recover. I would recommend that women take the time they need to recover. I found that it was uncomfortable to sit at work – there was pressure on the lower stomach region, which is where the stitches were located. After the third day, I was getting back into work but still felt a little winded and tired."

See the different ways hysterectomies are done

There's a fabulous medical animation company in the US called Nucleus Medical Media. It produces many of the animations you see on the *Dr. Oz Show*. If you go to my website, unhysterectomy. com, you can watch one of Nucleus's videos showing the difference between an abdominal, vaginal and laparoscopic hysterectomy. The video is produced for patients so it's short and easy to understand. Just like show and tell in elementary school, there's nothing like seeing something to really get a feel for what it's like. I highly recommend that you watch it before discussing all your options with your doctor, including the type of hysterectomy you may want if you go that route.

Chapter 7
The Perfect Storm: Why so Many Hysterectomies?

The number of hysterectomies being performed in Canada cannot be explained by any one factor. The issue is very complex. It would be too easy to blame doctors, or hospitals, or politicians or even women themselves for not demanding better care. At the end of the day, it's all those things and more.

In a nutshell, there is a perfect storm brewing in Canada that has swept women up in its path.

THE PERFECT STORM

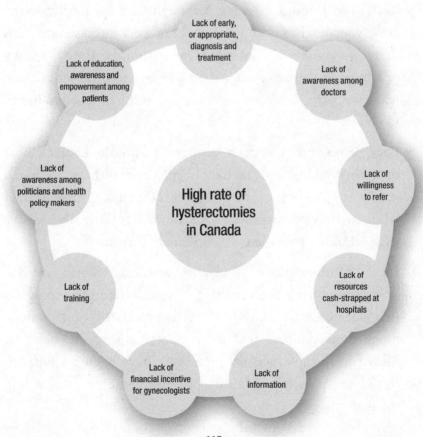

Canada's high hysterectomy rate attributable to many things

- **Lack of early, or appropriate is, diagnosis and treatment.** By the time a woman is finally seen by a gynecologist or given the proper diagnosis, she has usually seen a variety of physicians and is so physically, mentally and emotionally exhausted that she will often accept the first, most readily accessible and most permanent solution, which is usually hysterectomy.

- **Lack of awareness among doctors.** Some family physicians, and even some gynecologists, are not aware of some of the minimally invasive alternatives to hysterectomy that are available nowadays.

- **Lack of willingness to refer.** Although most family physicians and gynecologists have their patients' best interests at heart, there are those who, for whatever reason, be it ego, money or whatever, refuse to refer their patients to other physicians who can perform less-invasive surgeries. It happened to me so I know.

- **Lack of resources at cash-strapped hospitals.** Under global operating budgets, Canadian hospitals only have so much money to spend on all the procedures that must be performed within their operating rooms. Additionally, minimally invasive surgical suites are expensive and rare in Canada.

- **Lack of information.** Many, if not most, women are not being told during their initial visits with their gynecologists that options other than hysterectomy exist. Unfortunately, many gynecologists will offer only the surgery they feel most comfortable performing. There have been attempts in the US to pass laws making pre-hysterectomy counselling mandatory.

- **Lack of financial incentive**. As I mentioned earlier, gynecologists earn twice as much for performing an abdominal hysterectomy as they do for less invasive but more time-consuming and intricate surgery, such as endometrial ablation (see Chapter 13), that requires greater skill. Surgical fees are out of date and have not kept pace with technology or reality. This needs to change.

- **Lack of training**. Gynecologists, new and experienced, young and old alike, are struggling to embrace new technology and upgrade their surgical skills. Older gynecologists may not want to learn these newer procedures if they're close to retirement or if they're simply more comfortable with a scalpel in their hand than a laparoscope. Even some new graduates report feeling less than comfortable performing newer procedures.[70]

- **Lack of awareness among politicians and health policy makers** of the mental, physical, emotional, financial and societal benefits of minimally invasive surgery for women. Treatment of HMB is not even on the political radar in this country, never mind being targeted for improvement.

- **Lack of education, awareness and empowerment among patients** like you and me regarding alternatives to hysterectomy.

Many women I know chose to have a hysterectomy in about two seconds flat while others took months, if not years, to decide. The process of deciding whether to have the operation, whether or not we've had or will have children, is loaded with emotion and influenced by many things, not the least of which is other women's experiences.

---

[70] Jamie Kroft, Joel Moody and Patricia Lee, "Canadian Hysterectomy Educational Experience: Survey of Recent Graduates in Obstetrics and Gynecology," *Journal of Minimally Invasive Gynecology* 18, no. 4 (July 2011): 438-44.

Joyce posted this comment on my Facebook page. I could feel her suffering coming through the computer.

> I've been diagnosed with both endometriosis and adenomyosis, although I'm not sure it's possible to have both at the same time. I had a laparoscopy done for the endometriosis with one doctor and felt like she wasn't taking my pain seriously enough after the surgery. So I'm with a new doctor, who diagnosed the adenomyosis via MRI and has told me hysterectomy is the only option left.
>
> My appointment for the follow-up before scheduling surgery is this week. I've hit panic mode and just came across your site while doing research.
>
> I'm 26 years old. I was diagnosed in 2010. After I had my daughter via C-section in 2008 I kept getting more and more ill as time passed. No one knew of my endometriosis when I had my daughter and I was put on the birth control patch after I had her. Since then it's been hell trying to get something done about the pain I'm in. At first it was pain killers but the only thing that takes the pain away is OxyContin or Tylenol 3 and that was not an enjoyable experience. I feel like there really isn't enough push in the medical industry to search for alternative therapies instead of going straight for invasive, potentially harmful surgery. Don't get me wrong. I want the hysterectomy just to get rid of this pain. But I wish it didn't have to be this way.

I really hope Joyce finds the relief she needs through her upcoming hysterectomy. It's so sad that she has been forced to choose between preserving her fertility or ending her pain. Joyce mentioned she found me while doing research and I cannot overstate the importance of becoming more knowledgeable about hysterectomy and its alternatives.

Canadian writer Lise Cloutier-Steele's *Misinformed Consent: Women's Stories About Unnecessary Hysterectomy* is a poignant, yet disturbing, reminder of what can go wrong during surgery and of how the procedure affects some women. CBC Television's *Sex, Lies and Secrecy: Dissecting Hysterectomy* explores Canada's high hysterectomy rate and the negative after-effects that can be a consequence of this life-altering operation. CTV's *W-FIVE* feature *The Right to Know* chronicled the stories of 34 women who alleged that Toronto-area gynecologist Dr. Richard Austin maimed them during their surgeries. I remembering watching this documentary on TV back in 2008, two months after my surgery, and crying for these women whose lives were forever altered by their procedures. Even as I write, another Canadian gynecologist has been accused of the same kind of breach in southern Ontario.

The media and the Internet are full of stories about things gone wrong during surgery, not just hysterectomies. Our courts are full of patients wanting justice for one alleged infraction after another. The challenge for you and me, as women and potential patients, is to wade through these accounts and make the most informed choice possible. I urge you to read these books and watch these documentaries to gain a better understanding of both sides of the hysterectomy issue. Unfortunately, many women give their consent without fully understanding what it is they're signing up for. Here are the legal precedents, which I encourage you to read carefully:

"In obtaining the consent of a patient for the performance upon [the patient] of a surgical operation, a surgeon, generally, should answer any specific questions posed by the patient as to the risks involved and should, without being questioned, disclose to [the patient] the nature of the proposed operation, its gravity, any material risks and any special or unusual risks attendant upon the performance of the operation."[71] "...[A] surgeon must also, where the circumstances require it, explain to the patient the

---

[71] Supreme Court of Canada, Hopp v. Lepp, 1980.

consequences of leaving the ailment untreated and alternative means of treatment and their risks."[72]

That raises another interesting point, which is *informed refusal*. Our right to refuse treatment is enshrined in law. We have the right to refuse treatment if we desire, yet many of us automatically assume that if our doctor says we need a hysterectomy, we have to have one. Beware, however, that if you refuse treatment without a backup plan, your symptoms may continue. Another legal position:

"The right to determine what shall, or shall not, be done with one's own body, and to be free from non-consensual medical treatment, is a right deeply rooted in our common law. This right underlines the doctrine of informed consent. With very limited exceptions, every person's body is considered inviolate, and, accordingly, every competent adult has the right to be free from unwanted medical treatment. The fact that serious risks or consequences may result from a refusal of medical treatment does not vitiate the right of medical self-determination. The doctrine of informed consent ensures the freedom of individuals to make choices about their medical care. It is the patient, not the physician, who ultimately must decide if treatment – any treatment – is to be administered."[73]

Who you see is what you get

Hysterectomy rates across Canada vary widely. Although rates have been steadily declining over the past 20 years, the difference in rates across the country is troubling. In its *Health Indicators 2010* study, the Canadian Institute for Health Information (CIHI), which has been tracking hysterectomy rates since 2001, found that

---

[72] Saskatchewan Court of Appeal, Haughian v. Paine, 1987.
[73] Justice Sydney Robins, Ontario Court of Appeal, Fleming v. Reid, 1991.

rates in 2008-09 varied by more than 60 percent among provinces (after adjusting for population age differences). Rates ranged from a high of 512 per 100,000 women (age 20 or older) in Prince Edward Island to a low of 311 per 100,000 in British Columbia. Even more staggering was the fact that rates for rural women were *46 percent* higher than for urban women.[74]

"The differences in hysterectomy rates for menstrual disorders between urban and rural Canada may point to differences in clinical practice, rather than health differences," said Dr. Vyta Senikas, associate executive vice-president of the Society of Obstetricians and Gynecologists of Canada in a news release.[74]

Seven months later, the CIHI issued another report, *Health Care in Canada 2010*, which stated that care for certain conditions, including menstrual disorders, is not always appropriate and that "regional variations highlight potentially unnecessary surgical procedures."[75] John Wright, CIHI's president and CEO, weighed in: "Evidence and appropriateness of care are a significant issue in Canada's health care debate. The Organisation for Economic Co-operation and Development estimates that improving the efficiency of a public health system could save up to two percent of Gross Domestic Product. One way to improve system efficiency is to ensure the care provided is appropriate, based on the best available evidence."

My friend Mary, who suffered for years from crippling anemia and tremendously heavy flow, is a perfect example of what can happen when care is inconsistent. She received different opinions from two gynecologists in the same office in Ottawa. One wanted

---

[74] Canadian Institute for Health Information, "Heart Attacks More Likely among Lower-Income Groups, but Quality of Care about the Same for All Canadians," News release (May 27, 2010).

[75] Canadian Institute for Health Information, "Health Care in Canada 2010: Evidence of Progress, but Care Not Always Appropriate," 2010, http://www.cihi.ca/CIHI-ext-portal/internet/en/Document/health+system+performance/indicators/performance/RELEASE_16DEC10.

her to have a hysterectomy, while the other wanted her to have an endometrial ablation (discussed in Chapter 13). "Here I was worrying about how hysterectomy would affect my body and my femininity and these two gynecologists were disagreeing over whether or not to even do one. It didn't exactly help my confidence," recalls Mary.

Hysterectomy rates are just as varied around the world. "A disturbing issue, difficult to research but clamouring nevertheless for the research to be done, is the varying hysterectomy rate between countries, between regions within the same country, and indeed between gynecologists in the same hospital!" say Drs. Isaac T. Manyonda and Essam Hadoura of St. George's Hospital in London, England. "Could it be that where rates are low, women are being denied a highly effective operation? Conversely, where rates are high, are women being subjected to unnecessary operations? What is the ideal hysterectomy rate anyway? These are urgent issues that require careful research and protocols to attempt to resolve the controversies."[76]

Kira Leeb, CIHI's director of health systems performance, says it's almost impossible to establish appropriate rates, or benchmarks, for hysterectomy, or for many other types of surgery for that matter.

"There aren't a lot of procedures in Canada that have a benchmark associated with them, an identified absolute target that we should be reaching. Even the benchmark for Caesarean sections is between five and 15 percent, which is a huge range.

"In Canada, we have practice-based, evidence-based guidelines and we have recommendations. And so again, when we see

[76] Isaac T. Manyonda and Essam Hadoura, "Total Abdominal Hysterectomy," *Modern Management of Abnormal Uterine Bleeding* (London, UK: Informa Health Care, 2008), 277.

such wide variations, even with these evidence-based practice guidelines, that's again a question for us to start looking at what's going on and why there are so many differences. So it's very hard to determine a benchmark for a clinical or a surgical procedure. You really do have to do chart reviews and almost examine each individual case and decide what makes sense. So it's very challenging. It's much easier to look at who's doing what and under what circumstances and start to evaluate it that way."

So how can we, as patients, know if our gynecologists are truly giving us the right treatment in the right place at the right time? In 2009, Dr. Singh and Dr. Philippe Y. Laberge of the Department of Obstetrics and Gynecology, Centre Hospitalier de l'Université Laval in Quebec City, recognized that something had to change.

"In response to public demand and for greater health care accountability, the establishment of quality indicators in gynecology at the local and national level must be addressed immediately," they wrote in the *Journal of Obstetrics and Gynecology.*[77] Not only were Drs. Singh and Laberge concerned about the wide variation in hysterectomy rates across Canada, they were also concerned that despite national evidence-based guidelines set by SOGC recommending vaginal or laparoscopic hysterectomies, far too many gynecologists were still performing them abdominally. The doctors proposed using an index called "technicity," a system developed in France to compare the performance of hospitals across the country. Technicity is defined by the number of hysterectomies performed vaginally and laparoscopically divided by the total number of hysterectomies performed annually in a single department.

---

[77] Philippe Y. Laberge and Sukhbir S. Singh, "Surgical Approach to Hysterectomy: Introducing the Concept of Technicity," *Journal of Obstetrics and Gynaecology Canada* 31, no. 11 (2009): 1050-3.

"We have developed this scoring system to demonstrate the advantages of less-invasive surgical approaches, thereby supporting the concept of technicity and its relevance to practice," the doctors wrote. "Using technicity, gynecologists throughout Canada can monitor their shift towards minimally invasive procedures for hysterectomy, for the benefit of patients and society." Their argument? That based on these five indicators – duration of surgery, length of hospital stay, complication rate, hospital cost and quality of life – many studies over the past 20 years have shown that vaginal and laparoscopic hysterectomies are simply better for patients than abdominal ones. The doctors concluded their report by saying, "resources should be allocated to provide a structured and national effort to promote and teach vaginal and laparoscopic hysterectomy so that we move towards a higher technicity index."[78]

But what exactly is technicity?

"Technicity is really about what percentage of hysterectomies are being offered in the least invasive fashion," says Dr. Nicholas Leyland of the Society of Minimally Invasive Gynecology. "We would like to see the abdominal hysterectomy rate to be about 20 percent of the cases. And in many places across Canada it's up to 80 percent.

"When you look at procedures in all kinds of specialties, you do find this disparity. And this is something that I think we, as a medical profession, really have to address because the variation in standards of what is offered to patients in hysterectomy or in cardiac surgery and these sorts of things, are not really a function of disease disparity within our society. It really is a function of many factors, but in particular the training and the availability of technology and a lot of other issues. So I would venture to say that we as a medical profession have a lot of explaining to do."

---

[78] Philippe Y. Laberge and Sukhbir S. Singh, "Surgical Approach to Hysterectomy: Introducing the Concept of Technicity," *Journal of Obstetrics and Gynaecology Canada* 31, no. 11 (2009): 1050-3.

One of the factors that may influence the rate at which technicity is adopted is the potential for personal bias that many gynecologists bring to the table. Humans are creatures of habit and gynecologists are human. The majority of gynecologists in Canada (and the US) are still prescribing hysterectomy because it's what they were taught in medical school, it's what they're most comfortable performing and it pays more than less-invasive surgery. But although hysterectomy may work, is it appropriate in every case?

"In recent years, effective alternatives to hysterectomy have emerged, and these include both medical and surgical options. However, a dramatic reduction in hysterectomy rates has yet to materialize, perhaps bearing testimony to the efficacy of hysterectomy and/or the fact that habits die hard among gynecologists," say Drs. Manyonda and Hadoura.

Old habits appear to die hard even among younger gynecologists. A study published in the *Journal of Minimally Invasive Gynecology* in November 2010 measured the comfort level of new graduates in performing various types of hysterectomy. You would think that young, enthusiastic new graduates would want to embrace new technology and try for less-invasive surgeries. What the study found, however, is that "although laparoscopic hysterectomy has substantial benefits compared to an abdominal hysterectomy, Canadian residents in obstetrics and gynecology are not receiving adequate training to feel comfortable using the laparoscopic approach as opposed to the vaginal and abdominal routes. To improve patient care, further educational initiatives are needed to ensure that graduates are capable of performing all types of hysterectomy."[79]

---

[79] Jamie Kroft, Joel Moody and Patricia Lee, "Canadian Hysterectomy Educational Experience: Survey of Recent Graduates in Obstetrics and Gynecology," *Journal of Minimally Invasive Gynecology* 18, no. 4 (July 2011): 438-44.

I recently spoke with one of these new graduates at a major Canadian teaching hospital; she asked not to be identified. At 30, now in a practice of her own, she has a very interesting perspective on which type of hysterectomies are "appropriate."

> It's an interesting evolution. When I was in residency in Canada, if someone had asked me if I was training to be a laparoscopic surgeon, I would have said yes. But since graduating and going to conferences abroad and speaking to other surgeons from other places, I learned that [gynecologists in other countries] are doing much more difficult cases laparoscopically than I was doing at home.

> As a resident, you don't see a lot of follow-up with your patients so it's hard to get a perspective on which type of hysterectomy is appropriate. You're trained to do the procedures, you look after people in hospital, and the minute they leave, it's like, "Bye-bye, have a nice time." When you have your own practice, as I do now, you start seeing people [who have had abdominal hysterectomies] come back to see you. You see them for their check-ups after six weeks, then 12 weeks, then six months and a year, but then you start to see them coming in with complications or concerns. You did everything exactly the way they taught you to in residency, so you fixed Problem A, but now you see them coming back with Problem B.

> A lot of what I was seeing was people having pain issues because they had laparotomies (abdominal hysterectomies), who were de-compensating physically because they were unable to be active or unable to continue their normal activities. So I started wondering if there was a better way to do this. Given the level of laparoscopic skill I already had, it just required a little bit extra in order to do that. So I started pursuing various courses in the US, various conferences and things to learn new skills. And as I incorporated those into my practice, it was self-reinforcing. The people that I performed minimally invasive procedures on did better, they were happier, and ironically, I saw them less because Problem A was fixed and they didn't develop Problem B. So their existence was much better.

Does that mean that the onus is on individual gynecologists to learn newer techniques? Pretty much. The question is, do they?

According to Dr. David Toub, a gynecologist in Wyncote, Pennsylvania, and medical director of Gynesonics, a US medical device company that has created a new device for zapping fibroids called VizAblate (approved for use in Europe but not yet in Canada or the US), many gynecologists simply prefer working with scalpels than with scopes. He calls it "the glamour factor."

We're still seeing the glamour factor with abdominal hysterectomy and the ease factor. You're working with your hands and it's a standard, predictable operation that surgeons are used to. People do things that work for them. For a lot of surgeons, abdominal hysterectomy is something they're used to, they're comfortable with and if the patient doesn't object, why would they think otherwise unless they're focused on providing various options?

Now at the same time I don't want to give the impression that I think that anyone who does a hysterectomy is guilty of malpractice or hates women. I've done more than my share of hysterectomies. It is still a good operation. In many cases, particularly women with chronic pelvic pain or very severe bleeding that has not been able to be treated with less - with more conservative means, a hysterectomy can restore their quality of life and that's been shown in the literature and anecdotally. However, I think there's a difference between offering women options and their choosing a hysterectomy and performing it as a competent surgeon, and just telling a woman, "I only can do hysterectomy here" when other options exist.

There is still this attitude that once a woman is done with her childbearing her uterus is inconsequential. As a resident, I wasn't trained to particularly conserve the uterus unless the woman wanted fertility. It just wasn't part of our culture. I think that's changed a bit but we have a long way to go. Those of us who are passionate about minimally invasive gynecology now have it in our DNA but our challenge is to find a way to get that mindset into the general surgical community, the general gynecologist.

The anonymous young gynecologist I spoke with has indeed adopted that mindset but ultimately, she says, her colleagues, her hospital and our healthcare system aren't ready to hear it.

We all went into medical school to help people. I swore to do no harm. But if you're looking at traditional healthcare, where it's a bit like a sausage factory, it's all about how fast you can get everybody through the system. Not everybody gets the best treatment, but we're aiming for good enough for large numbers of people. Someone's got to pay the price for that.

It's sad to say but sometimes I get a lot of flak for doing something new, for doing something that the system doesn't perceive as "normal." If I perform new procedures such as laparoscopic hysterectomy or [other laparoscopic surgeries that will preserve a woman's uterus], everyone on the team, including my physician and nursing colleagues, have to learn how to use the equipment, they have to learn how to do these new procedures, they have to train people to understand what it is that we're doing for the patient.

And you know, it's a bit of an annoyance. It's annoying when they don't know the equipment. It's annoying when we don't have a piece of equipment or they don't know where to find it. You get the irritation factor from the booking office saying, "Well, you know, you can only book three cases today. Normally I would let you book five, but you're going to take extra time with this and we can't have you going overtime." You get the annoyance factor from your anesthesia colleagues saying, "Well, I've never done anything in this position before. Why would you have to keep her asleep longer? What is the point of doing this?" And you say, "Well, my patient will feel better, she'll go home sooner, she'll go back to her life sooner." But none of these people see patients outside the hospital. It's like being a resident again. Once the patient leaves the OR space, they're out of their consciousness. They don't care. Let me rephrase that. It's not that they don't care, but it doesn't personally impact them, right? The argument I have to keep making is that my patient will feel better.

When I tell my husband about the way my day went, and he, being a complete layperson, says, "Wait a minute, hold up. Excuse me?" And then I think about it and say, "Yeah, I guess that's kind of not great." So you know, when you're treading water in the middle of the ocean, you lose perspective of where you can be. It's not that the system doesn't care. I mean, everybody working in the system cares. The problem is what the patient wants and needs is not even on their radar anymore. I think sometimes patients are getting lost in the shuffle.

Dr. Allaire says that while laparoscopic surgery is certainly good for some patients, it can definitely take longer than traditional surgery, which, in turn, can tip the balance between benefits and risks. In medicine, that has to be the first concern, regardless of the method used.

"Even though an abdominal cut might take a bit longer to recover from, if a woman is requiring so much longer under anesthetic, in a head-down position with all the swelling that goes with that, the potential risks of being under so long are definitely a factor. There has to be a balance. I think women should respect their doctors for the knowledge and training and experience they have, but they should also balance that with the fact that they are smart, educated women. It can't be either/or. It has to be a conversation."

I am the first one to encourage women to have more informed conversations with their gynecologists. That's what this book is all about. But we, as women, must challenge our gynecologists on the potential biases they may bring to the conversation in the first place. How long have they been in practice? How many hysterectomies have they performed? Which type? Have they had training in laparoscopic or vaginal hysterectomies, or some of the newer alternatives? What is their philosophy of care?

I asked Dr. Leyland about the first gynecologist I saw who refused to refer me to Dr. Singh for less-invasive surgery. His answer surprised me.

"I've said frequently that, in medicine, who you see is what you get. So that particular physician really only had a few tools in his toolbox to be able to offer you as a patient. And unfortunately, his training was probably somewhat out of date, and he hadn't kept up with all the new options. And even if physicians are aware of the options, unfortunately they're not really explaining those completely to their patients. So it has to do with a very important issue, and that is fully informed consent. So if you're going to a physician and he suggests a hysterectomy, he really does have to offer you the whole breadth and depth of all the other different options. And even if he or she does not perform them, he or she should – if they are appropriate – refer the patient to another physician who may offer them." (By the way, as an aside, I recently contacted the first gynecologist I saw to find out why he refused to refer me to another gynecologist and to give him the opportunity to be interviewed for this book. His secretary put me on hold for about 10 minutes, finally coming back on the line with a simple "He doesn't have time for this.")

Ethics

For me, the issue is really about ethics. Was it unethical of my first gynecologist to refuse to refer me to another gynecologist? Maybe yes, maybe no. There are four basic principles to medical ethics, which, in my opinion, are more grey than black and white:

- **Respect for the autonomy of the patient**. Allowing patients to decide what to do with their bodies even if it appears to be medically wrong

- **Beneficence**. Promoting what is best for patients in order to help them

- **Non-maleficence**. Vowing to do no harm

- **Justice**. Equal access to care for patients

The principle of justice can be complicated. "Resources are limited; you cannot cure everybody and so priorities must be set (hence the notion of triage). In allocating care, the Justice principle holds that patients in similar situations should have access to the same care, and that in allocating resources to one group we should assess the impact of this choice on others. In effect, is what the patient is asking for fair? Will it lead to a burden to others (such as the family caregivers)? While your primary duty is to your patient, others will be affected by your decisions and there may be a tension between beneficence, autonomy and justice."[80]

At the end of the day, I got the surgery I wanted but not through the actions of any of my earlier physicians. Did my first gynecologist harm me or do an injustice? Did he fail to respect my right to choose? By the letter of the law perhaps not, but he certainly didn't help me, either.

Far too many women are trapped in this grey zone and have no real recourse, except to keep on trucking, women like Lisa from Prince Edward Island. After waiting four years to find a family physician and a gynecologist who could diagnose her pain and heavy bleeding, and undergoing an unexpected surgery to remove an intrauterine device that had somehow grown into one of her fibroids, Lisa found herself arguing with her gynecologist over the best course of action. It was the last thing she needed.

> On my follow-up visit I asked the doctor what could be done about my fibroid and she said a hysterectomy was the only suggestion. At that time she accidentally disclosed that I also had a growth on my ovary. When I asked about it, she just brushed my question off. Her answer was to have a hysterectomy. I said that I had no interest in this and that there must be another way. She simply said no, and said she was done with me if I didn't want the hysterectomy. So I suffered again and tried to find myself another referral.
>
> I finally got a referral to another doctor and waited many more months for an ultrasound. This doctor suggested a myomectomy [the fibroid is

---

[80] University of Ottawa, "Society, the Individual and Medicine. Basic Ethical Principles," 2012, www.med.uottawa.ca/sim/data/Ethics_e.htm.

removed through the abdomen], but she said that she couldn't promise that a full hysterectomy wouldn't happen once we were in the operating room. I asked for a referral to a woman's centre to weigh my options. She didn't seem happy about it but she was very professional. I have my first appointment in Halifax in January. My hope is to get rid of these huge fibroids, which are causing major pain and problems in my life, but at least I will have my body intact.

Unless we have ethics police standing outside doctors' offices asking, "Did you find everything you were looking for today?" it's buyer beware. But remember, hysterectomy remains the *only* definitive cure for HMB, for now, but it's irreversible. Please keep that in mind as you research the options you feel are right for you.

Chapter 8
To Remove or Not to Remove Your Ovaries

My friend Rhonda is a thyroid cancer survivor and one of those friends I grew up with in Downsview. She and I were thick as thieves in school and we're still friends to this day. Her Jewish humour can slay me to the ground in a heartbeat and leave us both weeping. One of the expressions she learned from her mother and passed on to me is one that many Jewish people say after someone says something that promises good things: "From your lips to God's ears." I love that expression. Whether it's winning the lottery, surviving cancer or passing an exam at university, we can try to attract good things in life just by saying them out loud so God, or whatever higher power you believe in, can hear our plea.

So from my lips to God's ears, I hope we find a cure for ovarian cancer.

Of all gynecological cancers, ovarian cancer is the most serious.[81] According to Ovarian Cancer Canada, more than 2,600 Canadian women are diagnosed and 1,750 women die from the disease every year. Ovarian cancer can be hard to detect because the symptoms are not that obvious and are often missed. There is no screening test to detect it, but if found early, ovarian cancer has a survival rate of 90 percent.

> In the past, many people assumed that as women go through menopause their ovaries turn off like a light switch. [We now know] that's not quite the case. There is a major decrease in estrogen production, but it's really a very slow, gradual diminution thereafter. It's not a complete on and off switch.
>
> – Dr. Jonathan Berek, Professor of Obstetrics and Gynecology – Gynecologic Oncology – Stanford University School of Medicine

---

[81] Ovarian Cancer Canada, "Knowledge and Awareness," 2012, www.ovariancanada.org.

What does ovarian cancer have to do with hysterectomy?

Aside from the obvious – that women diagnosed with ovarian cancer will usually have their ovaries removed – many women *at risk* for the disease will also have their ovaries removed as a preventive measure. This is called a prophylactic oophorectomy. While ovary removal is certainly understandable for women who have ovarian cancer or who are at high risk because they have a family history of the disease or they carry the breast cancer gene (BRCA), **most women who undergo oophorectomies are not at increased risk**. Their ovaries are removed "just in case." As mentioned, Canadian statistics are hard to find, but of the 600,000 or so hysterectomies performed in the US every year, about 300,000 include ovary removal and there are reasons to believe the Canadian experience is about the same, relatively speaking. Visit Ovarian Cancer Canada for a list of risk factors at ovariancanada.org.

Why are the numbers so high? Because that's what gynecologists have been taught to do for the past 60 plus years or so. According to the gynecologists I have spoken with, women over 40 undergoing hysterectomy for benign conditions were routinely encouraged to have their ovaries removed to prevent them from developing ovarian cancer. Yet statistically, ovarian cancer is not common, affecting only one in 70 women. But until recently, ovary removal has been standard procedure.

"For many years, doctors were taught that it's better to take the ovaries out because we all know how horrible it is to get ovarian cancer. By the time most women are diagnosed, they have advanced ovarian cancer and many will die," says Dr. Jonathan Berek, professor of obstetrics and gynecology and gynecologic oncology at Stanford University School of Medicine in Stanford, California.

In 2009, Dr. Berek, Dr. Parker and several colleagues published a landmark study[82] that found that removing a woman's ovaries might increase her risk of developing heart disease, lung cancer and other serious conditions. The study examined 29,380 women, 16,345 of whom had both ovaries removed during hysterectomy and 13,035 who retained their ovaries during hysterectomy. Researchers evaluated the disease and death rates among those women from heart disease, stroke, breast cancer, ovarian cancer, lung cancer, colorectal cancer, all cancers, hip fracture, pulmonary embolus (obstruction of the arteries in the lungs, often caused by blood clots) and death from all causes.

What they found is that removing ovaries in women at average risk of ovarian cancer did not reduce death rates overall, but rather led to a higher risk of death from cardiovascular disease and coronary artery disease, particularly in premenopausal women. Researchers also discovered that among women who had their ovaries removed, there was a 30 percent increase in deaths from lung cancer.

As well, in 2009, Dr. Anita Koushik, a researcher at the Université de Montréal's Department of Social and Preventive Medicine, found that women who experienced non-natural menopause through ovary removal are at almost twice the risk of developing lung cancer as women who experienced natural menopause.[83]

"When you start looking at long-term benefits and risk, it may be that preservation of ovarian function is better in many individuals. These are fairly recent studies so further examination is required," Dr. Berek told me. "But still, it's a major paradigm shift."

---

[82] W.H. Parker, M.S. Broder, E. Chang, D. Feskanich, C. Farquhar, Z. Liu, D. Shoupe et al., "Ovarian Conservation at the Time of Hysterectomy and Long-Term Health Outcomes in the Nurses' Health Study," *Obstetrics and Gynecology* 113, no. 5 (2009): 1027-37.

[83] Anita Koushik, "Characteristics of Menstruation and Pregnancy and the Risk of Lung Cancer in Women," *International Journal of Cancer* 125, no. 10 (Nov. 2009): 2428-33.

A year later, Dr. Parker, Dr. Berek and their colleagues released a follow-up study[84] strongly encouraging women who do not have the breast cancer gene or a family history of ovarian cancer to consider keeping their ovaries, especially if they have not yet reached menopause.

"So clearly, if you take the ovaries out, you don't get ovarian cancer. But it turns out that over the 24 years of the study, only 34 women died of ovarian cancer. There's no doubt ovarian cancer is a terrible disease, but it doesn't affect many people. Heart disease kills 30 times more women a year than ovarian cancer and stroke kills probably three times more women a year than ovarian cancer. These are big numbers compared to the small number of women dying of ovarian cancer. So the benefits of keeping your ovaries are many," says Dr. Parker, the study's lead author.

What are the benefits of keeping your ovaries?

Before menopause, our ovaries produce a lot of estrogen and male hormones called androgens, including testosterone and androstenedione. These hormones keep our heart, bones and blood vessels healthy. After menopause, our ovaries produce less estrogen, but they do continue to produce androstenedione and testosterone, which are then converted into estrogen and continue to protect our vital organs, including our heart and lungs.

So even though we may think our ovaries aren't functioning past menopause, they are still sending a continuous flow of estrogen to protect our blood vessels. If you remove the ovaries, you lose the estrogen and the androgens, and therefore their benefits to the blood vessels and our vital organs. In spite of these studies, there

---

[84] J.S. Berek, E. Chalas, M. Edelson, D.H. Moore, W.M. Burke, W.A. Cliby and A. Berchuck, "Prophylactic and Risk-Reducing Bilateral Salpingo-oophorectomy: Recommendations Based on Risk of Ovarian Cancer," *Obstetrics and Gynecology* 116 (Sept. 2010): 733-43.

is still some debate within the medical community as to whether or not this is true. And if it is true, at what age do our ovaries stop producing these vital hormones, if ever? I have heard estimates ranging from age 60 all the way up to age 90.

Additionally, a study published in the December 2011 issue of *Obstetrics and Gynecology*[85] found that women who undergo pre-menopausal hysterectomy were at nearly a twofold increased risk for ovarian failure as compared with women with intact uteruses. "Although it is unresolved whether it is the surgery itself or the underlying condition leading to hysterectomy that is the cause of earlier ovarian failure, physicians and patients should take into account this possible sequela [a secondary consequence or result] when considering options for treatment of benign conditions of the uterus," the authors concluded.

He said, she said

As with most things in life, there are two sides to every story. A study released in 2011 by University of California gynecology professor Dr. Vanessa Jacoby[86] found that although removing both ovaries during hysterectomy did decrease the risk of ovarian cancer compared with keeping them, ovarian cancer was rare in both groups she studied. Her study further concluded that removing both ovaries "may not have an adverse effect on cardiovascular health, hip fracture, cancer, or total mortality compared with hysterectomy and ovarian conservation." The study looked at 25,448 post-menopausal women aged 50 to 79 with no history of ovarian cancer who either had their ovaries removed or preserved

---

[85] P. G. Moorman, E. Myers, Evanm J. Schildkraut, E. Iversen, F. Wang, N. Warren, "Effect of Hysterectomy With Ovarian Preservation on Ovarian Function," *Obstetrics & Gynecology* 118, no. 6 (Dec. 2011): 1271-1279.

[86] V. Jacoby, "Oophorectomy vs. Ovarian Conservation with Hysterectomy. Cardiovascular Disease, Hip Fracture, and Cancer in the Women's Health Initiative Observational Study," *Archives of Internal Medicine* 171, no. 8 (Apr. 2011): 768-9.

during their hysterectomies. The women were participating in the Women's Health Initiative study.[87]

As a layperson, I find these kinds of contradictory studies frustrating. On the one hand, they're informative and thought-provoking, but on the other hand, they're frightening and confusing. Who and what are we to believe? It's important to note that the ages of the women and the length of time they were followed varied in both of these studies. The women in Dr. Parker's study were younger (30–55) and were followed for a longer period of time (24 years). The women in Dr. Jacoby's study were older (around 63) and followed for only seven years so Dr. Jacoby's study conclusions are less clear-cut. It's a bit like comparing apples and oranges.

I think as the end users, or recipients, of this knowledge, we should use the information as a starting point, a way to open a discussion with our doctors about the best course of treatment for us, given our family history and our potential risk factors. Remember, unless you are at increased risk because of your history, the decision to remove your ovaries or not is entirely up to you, not your doctor.

"No longer should it be a one-way conversation from doctor to patient saying, 'I'm going to take out your ovaries' and the patient saying, 'OK,'" says Dr. Parker. "It has to be a conversation. What are your risk factors? Should we or shouldn't we remove your ovaries? It's no longer just a pat answer. I think it's a little more complicated and hopefully this latest research will change the conversation between women and their doctors."

---

[87] US National Institutes of Health, National Heart, Lung, and Blood Institute, 2010, www.nhlbi.nih.gov/whi/.

Some final food for thought

If we know a) that our ovaries continue to emit hormones that protect our hearts and lungs even after menopause, b) that surgically removing our ovaries increases our risk of heart disease and lung cancer, c) that heart disease and stroke are the leading cause of death in Canadian women[88] and that lung cancer is the leading cancer killer among women,[89] is it possible there is a connection between these three factors? I am no scientist, but I can't help but wonder if there is.

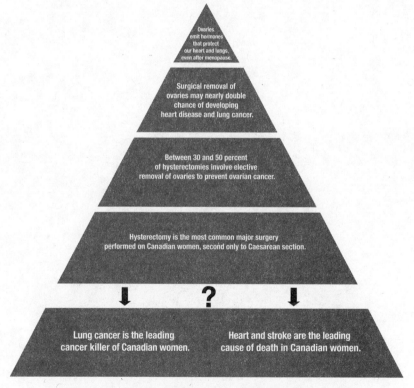

OVARY REMOVAL, HEART DISEASE AND LUNG CANCER:
IS THERE A CONNECTION?

---

[88] Heart and Stroke Foundation of Ontario, "Women and Heart Disease and Stroke," 2012, www.heartandstroke.on.ca.
[89] Canadian Cancer Society. "Lung Cancer Statistics at a Glance," 2012, www.cancer.ca.

Chapter 9
The XXX Factor: Hysterectomy and Sex

Ask a room full of women if their sex lives are better or worse after hysterectomy and I bet the room would be divided right down the middle. Some women I know are having great sex after their hysterectomies because their pain and bleeding are gone; some are having no sex at all; others are working on it.

Except for those rare, terrible cases in which women have been accidentally damaged during surgery and can no longer physically have vaginal sex, the number of women having good or bad sex after hysterectomy appears to be almost impossible to measure. Should we assume that the quality of their sex lives is related entirely to their surgery or are there other factors at play? How strong a sex drive did these women have before they started bleeding heavily? How did the bleeding affect their sex life? Did they care about sex before surgery? Did they care after? Are they having problems? Are they depressed? Anxious? Angry? If they had their ovaries removed, could menopause, or the fact that they may have gained weight, be lowering their sex drive? When do you ask these questions? After six weeks? Six months, a year, five years?

Perhaps all these unknowns are why scientists seem to be stumped, too. There doesn't seem to be any conclusive evidence one way or the other about whether hysterectomy affects women sexually. One study, published in the May 2011 issue of the *Journal of Minimally Invasive Gynecology*,[90] called "Hysterectomy Improves Sexual Response? Addressing a Crucial Omission in the

---

[90] Barry R. Komisaruk, Eleni Frangos and Beverly Whipple, "Hysterectomy Improves Sexual Response? Addressing a Crucial Omission in the Literature," Journal of Minimally Invasive Gynecology 18, no. 3 (May 2011): 288-95, www.jmig.org/article/PIIS155346501100015X/fulltext.

Literature," does raise some very interesting questions. I find the abstract particularly telling:

> The prevailing view in the literature is that hysterectomy improves the quality of life. This is based on claims that hysterectomy alleviates pain (dyspareunia [pain during sex] and abnormal bleeding) and improves sexual response.

> Because hysterectomy requires cutting the sensory nerves that supply the cervix and uterus, it is surprising that the reports of deleterious [harmful] effects on sexual response are so limited. However, almost all articles that we encountered report that some of the women in the studies claim that hysterectomy is detrimental to their sexual response.

> It is likely that the degree to which a woman's sexual response and pleasure are affected by hysterectomy depends not only on which nerves were severed by the surgery, but also the genital regions whose stimulation the woman enjoys for eliciting sexual response.

> Because clitoral sensation (via pudendal and genitofemoral nerves) should not be affected by hysterectomy, this surgery would not diminish sexual response in women who prefer clitoral stimulation. However, women whose preferred source of stimulation is vaginal or cervical would be more likely to experience a decrement in sensation and consequently sexual response after hysterectomy because the nerves that innervate [supply] those organs, that is, the pelvic, hypogastric, and vagus nerves, are more likely to be damaged or severed in the course of hysterectomy.

> However, all published reports of the effects of hysterectomy on sexual response that we encountered fail to specify the women's preferred sources of genital stimulation. As discussed in the present review, we believe that the critical lack of information as to women's preferred sources of genital stimulation is key to accounting for the discrepancies in the literature as to whether hysterectomy improves or attenuates sexual pleasure.

I think the "critical lack of information" they are referring to is asking, "What turns your crank?"

US sex therapist Dr. Laura Berman made some fascinating comments on *The Marlo Thomas Show*[91] in a piece called "A Hysterectomy's Effects on Libido, from Dr. Laura Berman." You can watch the episode online. A woman had written in to say things were not going very well in the bedroom since she had a partial hysterectomy and she wanted to know if hysterectomy can affect your libido.

"You know what? It can," said Dr. Berman. "For two reasons. One – and what she's saying is her libido and her ability to reach orgasm [are both affected]. So this is something that I know will annoy you in the way it annoys me: there are unbelievable amounts of anatomical research on men, on the crucial nerves and blood vessels that are essential to sexual function. They now go in with robotic little surgical machines to do prostate surgery on a man to make sure they're sparing every nerve. They haven't even mapped the nerves and blood vessels that are essential to a woman's sexual function that are all in our pelvis, so they just go in and cut and it's the luck of the draw, basically, whether you end up with sexual functioning or not, and the research kind of flushes that out post-hysterectomy."

> *Ever since I had my hysterectomy it's been a free-for-all. Bring it on, baby. Sex was so painful and a chore before, but now I'm free and having great, great, great sex.*
>
> – Paula, 51

Dr. Berman also said that if women are in tremendous pain and having heavy bleeding before their hysterectomy, then it stands to reason that their sex life would likely improve. But for women who have a hysterectomy for reasons that weren't necessarily affecting their sex lives before, then their sex lives might actually become worse. Because women climax clitorally, vaginally and through deep contractions coming from the pelvic floor and the

---

[91] Laura Berman, "Hysterectomy Effects on Libido," 2012, www.marlothomas.com.

uterus, surgically removing your uterus may lead to less-intense, less-enjoyable orgasms. Also, if your surgeon accidentally cuts any nerves or blood vessels that are essential to sensation, you could lose some sensitivity and ability to reach orgasm.

Calgary sex therapist Dr. Trina Read (trinaread.com) says that before we can even begin to understand the role hysterectomy might play in our sex drive we have to become more educated. Do you know the difference between sexual desire, libido and sexual arousal? Do you have vaginal, clitoral or G-spot orgasms, or none at all? In other words, what is your XXX Factor? Here's what Dr. Read says:

> *Although I chose not to have a hysterectomy, my sex life had been pretty much non-existent for years because of the pain and heavy bleeding.*
>
> *As soon as I hit menopause and stopped bleeding, I went out and bought myself the sexiest lingerie I could find. I even bought some crotchless underwear.*
>
> *- Tanya, 59*

Sexual desire is about the thoughts that go on in our head. And it's usually the number one reason why couples in North America stop having sex. I call it the "Oh crap phenomenon." "Oh crap, do I have to have sex tonight?" "Oh crap, is it time again?" And because we have negative thoughts going into the sexual experience, and for too many women, after the sexual experience, it just builds up a very negative feeling towards the act of sex. So I think when we're looking at something like a hysterectomy or heavy bleeding, there's that anxiety that goes along with the sexual experience that if you don't talk about it with your partner or if you don't acknowledge it, it's really, really going to impact your ability to have good thoughts and have good sex.

Libido is the hormones that we have in our body that naturally propel us to want to have sex. So women, especially when we're in our 20s, we're all juiced up with a nice balance of estrogen and progesterone. As we age, we're not as balanced in our hormones and when we start reaching peri-menopause, which is just before we go into menopause, our hormones are completely out of whack. So when we look at removing our ovaries, sometimes this balance of hormones goes out of whack [even further]. So not having a balance in your hormones is going to affect your want and desire to have sex.

Sexual arousal is the actual ability to get aroused during sex. So when we think about a man getting aroused, how do we know a man is aroused? Hmm. His penis moves from a flaccid state to an erect state. Something similar happens in a woman's body. When a man's penis is erect it engorges with blood. Now a woman has what's called an orgasmic platform, and it is a much, much bigger surface area. If you look at your entire pelvis area, that's your orgasmic platform. That entire platform must engorge with blood in order for your vulva [your external sex organs] to become properly aroused. The thing about your vulva is that when your vagina is in a resting state, it is a collapsed tube. When blood starts engorging the vaginal canal, it becomes a tube-like construction that starts to sweat and that's your lubrication.

Unfortunately for a lot of women, they do not become properly aroused. So her vulva and her vaginal canal do not become properly aroused before intercourse starts. And so that can have different implications where intercourse isn't as comfortable, she isn't as well-lubricated as she possibly can be, and it's just not the nicest experience. So when I talk to couples about when they used to be really excited about sex and having some of the best sex they ever had, inevitably the woman has been juiced up, completely aroused, and the intercourse was just amazing.

When we're looking at your sexuality after having a hysterectomy or if you're bleeding heavily, you have to sit down and say to yourself "OK, is it my sexual desire that's being affected? Is it my libido that's being affected? Or am I not being properly aroused when I go into that sexual experience?" It could be a combination of one or two or three and that can make or break the difference to you having good sex or having not so great sex.

What's a girl to do?

Go to my website and listen to my entire interview with Dr. Trina. She's got some great tips and tricks for getting in the mood, whether you've had a hysterectomy or not.

Take the study on sexual functioning I mentioned earlier and show it to your gynecologist. I'm sure he or she would be happy to answer any questions you might have about what it all means.

Diamonds aren't a girl's only best friend

The popularity of sex toys is on the rise around the world for mainstream couples wanting to spice things up between the sheets. In fact, according to a study released by Dr. Berman in 2004[92] one in five US women said they used self-stimulation at least once a week, and of those women, nearly 60 percent reported using a sex toy. Additionally, the study found that 44 percent of women between the ages of 18 and 60 have used a sexual device.

I wouldn't have been caught dead using a sex toy until I read a very interesting story on the front page of the *Ottawa Citizen* in January 2009 about a normal, average, everyday couple from little North Gower, Ontario – Bruce and Melody Murison – who invented a sex toy called the We-Vibe. Actually, Bruce invented it in his basement after being laid off from Nortel. To cut a long story short, in less than five years these very nice, very humble hockey parents have produced one of the hottest-selling sex toys in the world! They have sold more than a million We-Vibes, and do you know why?

"What can I say?" says Melody. "My husband is a genius." First of all, these things work. And second, you can actually wear the c-shaped We-Vibe while you make love so both of you can enjoy the sensation. One of the vibrating pads sits right over your clitoris while the other sits near your G-spot. The device is slim enough that your partner can enter and enjoy the throbbing sensations as well. There are nine different modes and strengths – the grandchild of We-Vibe, We-Vibe III, is 40 percent stronger than Bruce's original model. Because clitoral stimulation is so important to women

---

[92] Laura Berman, "The Health Benefits of Sexual Aids & Devices: A Comprehensive Study of their Relationship to Satisfaction and Quality of Life. New Study on Female Sexuality Reveals Increased Use of Sexual Aids by Women (The Berman Center, 2004).

who've had their uterus removed, the We-Vibe offers tremendous potential for stimulation.

If sex is important to you, and you want to experiment with new ways of discovering your XXX Factor, perhaps you should try a toy. The We-Vibe has been commented on by relationship therapists, sexual health experts and medical professionals around the world, including Dr. Read, Dr. Robin Milhausen (as featured on CBC's *Steven & Chris Show*) and others. We-Vibe II has been featured at scientific, medical and academic research conferences, including meetings of the Society for the Scientific Study of Sexuality; the American Association of Sexuality Educators, Counselors and Therapists; and The Guelph Sexuality Conference.

What have you got to lose?

PART IV

MINIMALLY INVASIVE
ALTERNATIVES TO HYSTERECTOMY

Chapter 10
Less Is More

The process of choosing to avoid a hysterectomy through less-invasive medical or surgical means is serious business. As I've mentioned, hysterectomy remains the only definitive cure for painful, heavy menstrual bleeding, so if you decide against it, be absolutely sure this is what you want. You can always change your mind down the road, but remember, wait times for any kind of surgery are long in Canada and you will have lost valuable time in the queue if you choose to go back in line.

The right to choose is a precious right so we should use it wisely. Dr. Singh says,

> The right to choose is a basic principle that men and women have around the world. The United Nations Charter of Human Rights stipulates we should have the ability to make decisions for ourselves and to vote. In Canada, that has also meant that you should be able to choose what to do with your body. It comes down to the abortion debate, infertility, reproduction or taking contraception.

> So for me, at the end of the day, if you're in a situation where you have heavy menstrual bleeding or big fibroids or lots of pain, and someone says you can only have a hysterectomy even though you would like to explore less-invasive ways of relieving your symptoms, that person is not giving you the right to choose and that's wrong.

> Many women end up choosing hysterectomy anyway by the time they see me because they're so fed up with suffering. They know we can perform less-invasive surgeries that will preserve their uterus, and I would do that if they asked me to, within reason, but they say, "Unless you can promise me that I'll never have another period I'm having the hysterectomy." The reason why I am so passionate about minimally invasive gynecology is that even when a woman does choose to have a hysterectomy, we can perform the surgery so much less invasively than through a deep abdominal cut. Minimally invasive surgery presents fewer risks and is simply better for the patient, whether you're doing a hysterectomy or not.

A lasting imprint

While I was interviewing Dr. Ashton for this book, she used a term that I believe aptly describes the weight of responsibility gynecologists carry when working with their patients. She used the term *fingerprints*.

Some people really couldn't care less whether they take out their appendix, their gallbladder, their uterus, or their this or their that. They don't care. But as a surgeon, I am very aware of the fingerprints I leave on a patient. I have a responsibility not to develop tunnel vision or see things in isolation.

When I was doing abdominal surgery, I would always think to myself, "This patient is 45 now, but what about when she's 75?" What I leave now in terms of my fingerprints in this surgery is going to be relevant 30 years from now. So you can never do anything in a vacuum. And I think that that's a very, very important factor. It's very easy for a healthy 45-year-old woman to say, "Yes, I'm just going to have a hysterectomy," but if she's 75 and she has colon cancer, [she's going to have] scar tissue in her abdomen from a hysterectomy that might complicate the colon cancer surgery. So I think that there are a lot of angles that have to be looked at.

Does hysterectomy have to be performed in some cases? Absolutely. There are definitely times when a hysterectomy is appropriate. I have a patient right now who's 50 years old thinking she can delay surgery because she may go into menopause. Her uterus is 24 centimetres large. It's well above her belly button. So you know, at that point, I don't care if it's going to shrink 20 or 30 percent in menopause, it really needs to come out. I will likely refer her to one of my colleagues because since I started my full-time second career as the medical correspondent for CBS News, I stopped doing hysterectomies because I felt it was surgically inappropriate for me to perform these surgeries only once a year. So when a woman comes to me for a second opinion, I have no skin in the game. Whether she gets the surgery or not, I'm not going to get paid. So I'm there to explain to her all of the options and unfortunately many women are only told about the procedures their doctor can perform himself or herself, and that is unacceptable.

Before you make any decisions, Dr. Singh and Dr. Ashton recommend that you ask yourself five key questions:

- How bad are my symptoms?
- Are my symptoms affecting my quality of life?
- How old am I?
- Do I want to have children?
- What level of invasiveness am I comfortable with?

Your doctor may ask you the same questions so it's a good idea to have your answers ready.

Five benefits of minimally invasive surgery

1. It requires fewer incisions or no incisions at all, depending on the procedure.

2. It carries a lower risk of bladder or bowel perforation.

3. Some procedures can be done without general anesthetic.

4. Many minimally invasive procedures can be done as day surgery.

5. Recovery is faster, less painful and carries a lower risk of post-operative infection or complications.

Chapter 11
Watchful Waiting, Tranexamic Acid and Hormone Therapy

What I have prepared for you in the next four chapters is a summary of the main medical and surgical alternatives to hysterectomy that are available today in Canada and the United States. Again, this information is presented as a jumping off point to trigger a more in-depth conversation with your family doctor, gynecologist or other healthcare provider. The information is by no means exhaustive. It simply gives you an overview of the main options that are available.

With that in mind, there are three main medical treatments that doctors should try first, before prescribing anything more invasive: watchful waiting, tranexamic acid and hormone therapy.

Watchful waiting

Remember my friend Maureen, who suffered for seven years before finally reaching menopause? Although she saw her gynecologist throughout that time, she chose to monitor her symptoms through watchful waiting. She may not have known the term, but that's what doctors call the conscious choice that some women make to actively monitor their symptoms. Doctors are adamant about explaining the difference between watchful waiting and doing nothing. Doing nothing means just that. Watchful waiting, on the other hand, means keeping track of your symptoms and reporting any changes to your doctor. Many women choose watchful waiting until they can no longer live with their symptoms, sometimes for months or even years, as we saw with Maureen.

Thirty-two-year-old Melanie is a professional singer, dancer and actor who was uncomfortable with the idea of having a hysterectomy for a variety of reasons. Not only was she concerned about losing six weeks of work, she was also concerned about possible abdominal scarring and how that would affect her mobility on stage. So when an ultrasound revealed she had a fibroid the size of a 16-week pregnancy growing in her lower belly, she tried treating the mass on her own with natural alternatives. She tried watchful waiting for a while with naturopathy, hands-on energy healing from a Reiki master, meditation and herbal remedies, but nothing worked. After enduring "the worst day of my life," when she was told she needed a hysterectomy, Melanie inquired about less-invasive surgery.

The day she was scheduled to have a laparoscopic myomectomy, her surgeon fell ill and it was Dr. Singh who ended up performing the procedure. After a textbook recovery, Melanie is back dancing and performing and feeling great.

> I feel truly blessed. It was fate that Dr. Singh ended up performing the operation. Knowing my profession, he gave me the smallest incision, about the size of my thumb. I was in the Dominican Republic last month wearing a bikini and the scar was so small you couldn't even see it. Not that it was an issue for me cosmetically, it's just that certain costumes [are revealing]. He was amazing. I had no problems. The whole experience was wonderful compared to my earlier appointments, when the first doctor I met said, "Well, at your age, hysterectomy is really your only option." It was so harsh.
>
> My partner and I are non-traditionalists to begin with so we hadn't really thought about kids per se, but to discover that we might lose the opportunity was very emotional. Psychologically it destroyed me. Just hearing the word "hysterectomy" was horrendous for me. But then hearing there were options made me more determined than ever to go that route.
>
> It doesn't matter whether you're in your childbearing years or not, removing something that is natural to us is super-traumatic physically, emotionally and mentally. There are other options. So my advice to women is to explore all your options before making your decision. Make as informed a decision as possible that works for you and only you.

Like any treatment option, watchful waiting has advantages and disadvantages.

Advantages

- It's non-invasive.

- It buys you time.

- It may take you right up to menopause.

Disadvantages

- Just like your first period, menopause will come in its own sweet time. There's no way of knowing just when your period will stop.

- You may develop iron-deficiency anemia. Anemia (a low red-blood-cell count) affects the amount of oxygen circulating through your body, which affects the functioning of your vital organs. It can be dangerous if left untreated.

Non-hormonal medical options

Anti-inflammatories

Believe it or not, those pills you keep stashed in your purse for the occasional headache or menstrual cramp can actually help reduce your flow as well. When taken regularly (as soon as your period starts), medications like ibuprofen or naproxen (Advil, Motrin or Aleeve) can actually help reduce the volume of blood during your period (between 30 and 50 percent). The key is to take it regularly during your period.

Advantages

- It's cheap and easy to use.

- It will help with pain and bleeding.

Disadvantages

- It may cause some stomach upset (so take with food).
- It doesn't work for everyone.

Tranexamic acid

Tranexamic acid (Cyklokapron) belongs to a group of medicines called antifibrinolytic agents, which are prescribed to stop heavy bleeding or assist blood clotting. My family doctor prescribed Cyklokapron from the beginning, but I found it never really helped. I found out years later that I should have been taking it *as soon as I started bleeding* every month, so maybe I didn't take it at the right time. On my heaviest days, I took three or four tablets every four hours around the clock, yet I hardly noticed a difference.

Advantages

- Tranexamic acid is non-invasive and is taken by mouth. It can help reduce the heaviness of flow provided you take it *as soon as you start bleeding* and maintain the dose *your doctor prescribes*.

Disadvantages

- It may not reduce your flow.
- It does have possible side effects, which you should discuss with your doctor and your pharmacist.

Hormone therapy

Hormone therapy is often recommended as a first-line treatment for HMB. Doctors will often recommend either the birth control pill or progestins (synthetic progesterone).

Birth control pill

The most common hormonal treatment used for heavy bleeding is actually the birth control pill. It can be taken in pill form, as a patch or even as a ring inserted into the vagina every month. It will reduce bleeding significantly and protect against pregnancy as well.

Advantages

- It's easy to use.

- It provides contraception.

- It reduces the risk of ovarian cancer and endometrial cancer.

Disadvantages

- Side effects in some women include headaches, nausea, breast tenderness and spotting.

- There is a rare risk of blood clots (especially if you have a personal or family history of clots, if you smoke and are over 35 or have high blood pressure).

Progestins (synthetic progesterone)

Recall from Chapter 4 that progesterone is important in controlling your periods. But it's also available in different forms that can help control your heavy bleeding. Synthetic forms can be taken by mouth every day, by injection every three months or in an intrauterine device (IUD) (see next chapter).

Advantages

- It can be taken by women who want to avoid estrogen (for example, women at risk of blood clots or smokers over age 35).

- It's easy to take.

Disadvantages

- Side effects can be really annoying (weight gain, bloating and acne).

- The injection (also known and Depo-Provera) has been shown to affect your bones after just two years of using it. Talk to your doctor about this if you are on this medication for more than two years. Some women will be on it for longer without any problems so it really depends on each individual.

Danazol

Danazol lowers estrogen and increases androgen (a sex hormone present in low levels in women) levels. It puts your body into a state similar to menopause by stopping ovulation and shrinking uterine growths.

Advantages

- It's non-invasive.

- It significantly reduces bleeding and increases menstrual regularity.

Disadvantages

- It can cause weight gain, upper gastrointestinal upset, acne and irritability.

- It cannot be taken by women with liver disease.

Gonadotropin-releasing hormone analogue therapy

I always smile when I see the term "gonadotropin-releasing hormone analogue" (GnRH-a) because it makes me think of the word "gonads," a slang term many men use to refer to their testicles. But the root of the word gonadotropin is, in fact, "gonad," and it does indeed refers to the organs – testes in men and ovaries in women – that produce specific types of sex hormones.

Women produce two types of gonadotropins: follicle-stimulating hormone (FSH) and luteinizing hormone (LH). If you've ever gone for blood work to see how close you are to menopause, these are the hormones your doctor will test. As soon as these hormones are produced by your pituitary gland, gonadotropins trigger production of other sex hormones. Men and women need these hormones to produce eggs and sperm; they're also responsible for the development of female and male traits such as voice changes, muscle development, hair growth and breast development.

By changing the amount of gonadotropins in our bodies, we can stop our periods altogether, or enter menopause.

GnRH *analogue* refers to synthetic hormones known as agonists and antagonists. Some GnRH *analogues* are taken as nasal sprays while others are injected under the skin, either in the abdomen or the butt. These drugs can be used either to induce medical menopause or to increase fertility. Agonists act by attaching to receptors on the pituitary gland, which in turn triggers our bodies to produce more LH and FSH than normal at the beginning. This is known as the "flare effect" and can actually make things worse before it makes them better. But because these agonists don't let go of the receptors, the pituitary gland then temporarily shuts down, thereby preventing ovulation and menstruation. Gynecologists will often prescribe GnRH *agonist* injections for HMB as a way to thin the lining of the uterus and shrink fibroids before surgery.

There are three kinds of GnRH-a therapy your doctor may prescribe to prepare you for surgery or give you some temporary relief:

- **Goserelin acetate**, a pellet that's injected into the abdomen every 28 days

- **Leuprolide acetate**, injected into a muscle (usually your butt) in one-month or three-month doses

- **Nafarelin acetate**, a nasal spray you use twice a day

GnRH-a therapy can be a godsend (at least they were for me) because they stop your period dead in its tracks. Of course, these hormones throw your body into instant menopause. For women who are close to menopause and have already experienced a slow, gradual decline in FSH and LH, the transition to full menopause may not be that difficult. But for a younger woman such as Shannon, who was 30 at the time of her injections, the change can be almost unbearable. "My hair started falling out, my skin dried up, I was moody and irritable all the time. I was happy not to have my period anymore but I felt like I aged 20 years overnight."

Advantages

- It is minimally invasive.

- It will control your bleeding in the short term.

- It will bring you relief for three to six months.

Disadvantages

- GnRH-a treatment throws your body into *instant* menopause. Symptoms can include hot flashes, mood swings, vaginal dryness, decreased sexual interest, increased low-density lipoprotein (bad) cholesterol levels, decreased high-density lipoprotein (good) cholesterol levels, insomnia and headaches.

- The flare effect can result in severe and unexpected "flooding" episodes (as I had). Be on your guard and keep supplies and a change of clothes handy just in case. It will get better once the "flare" settles and your hormones turn off.

- The cost. These medications are quite expensive if you don't have a drug plan.

If the menopausal symptoms become too much, ask your gynecologist about "adding back" some hormones to help you cope. The "add back" is a touch of estrogen that can be given by mouth or through the skin; it gets rid of the side effects without causing your bleeding to return.

The medical treatment options we have just explored are viable alternatives if you're looking for non-surgical ways to manage your symptoms in the short and long term. Again, it's all about what's right for you, determined after discussing these options with your doctor.

Chapter 12
The Mirena IUD

The levonorgestrel intrauterine device, known as the Mirena IUD, has revolutionized the treatment of abnormal uterine bleeding. Health Canada first approved the Mirena IUD in 2000 as a birth control device and it has since been approved in Canada, the US and around the world as a treatment for HMB.

Since its launch, the Mirena IUD has been used by more than 12 million women worldwide for contraception, treatment of HMB and hormone replacement therapy (HRT), although it is not approved for use as HRT in Canada. The Mirena is a three-centimetre, T-shaped plastic device that is inserted through the cervix into the uterus. It contains enough hormone to stay in place for up to five years. It works by releasing small amounts of the synthetic sex hormone levonorgestrel into the uterus. Levonorgestrel is commonly used in combination with oral contraceptives and is similar to progesterone, the sex hormone our bodies produce on their own. I personally loved the Mirena. It relieved my heavy bleeding almost right away and although I spotted for a year, at that point I was just happy to be clot-free.

Remember Sherri, who has sticky blood syndrome? Her gynecologist prescribed the Mirena for her heavy

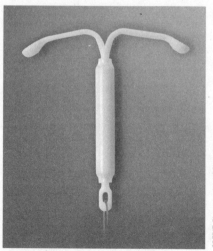

CREDIT: Photo courtesy ©Bayer Inc.

The levonorgestrel intrauterine device, known as the Mirena IUD.

bleeding and it worked like a charm. She chuckles when she thinks back to the day she went to pick it up from the drug store.

> So I go to Shoppers Drug Mart and I wait for the pharmacist to get it from the back and honest to God, he comes out with a box as long as a roll of wrapping paper. All I could think of was, "Is this going to fit inside of me?" Anyway, it went in OK with just a bit of a pinch but that night I had a dream that I was having a baby and that I had to push. I've never had a baby so it was weird that I wanted to keep pushing. I guess my brain was saying I had this thing inside of me. It wasn't painful or anything. I just knew there was something in there.

> Since that time it's performed just as the brochure says. I've had the textbook experience with the Mirena IUD. That was the end of September. I went back to see my doctor in November because I was spotting almost every day from October, November to mid-December. But he assured me it was normal and that by January it should stop. It pretty much did. I still get periods but it's been gradually reduced.

> So I'm sold on it because I know I don't want to have a stroke so I know I'm going to be on warfarin for the rest of my life. I had the Mirena put in when I was 44 and my doctor told me that it was good for five years, so with the anticipation that I'll be near menopause when I'm 49 I think it will be OK. It's amazing that I went from wearing a Depends, a tampon and two pads to wearing a pad a day, if that.

> I would just like to say to other women that the world of medicine nowadays is so progressive. If you have a problem and it's bothering you there is a solution out there. You may not know what it is and maybe your immediate doctors may not know what it is but there is something out there and you just have to find it.

Not all women have had the same kind of positive experience with the Mirena as Sherri. Our bodies are so unique that no two women will experience the same treatment the same way which is why it is so crucial to discuss your options with your doctor and pay very close attention to how your body feels throughout any form of treatment.

Time for show and tell

The success of the Mirena IUD in lightening or stopping HMB presents not only life-changing relief for many women, it also presents a unique learning opportunity for physicians. In 2010, Dr. Susan Phillips, a family physician and professor at Queen's University in Kingston, Ontario, had a hunch that family doctors were suffering from information overload and that maybe it was time for some good old-fashioned show and tell. Instead of *telling* doctors about the latest research showing how devices such as the Mirena IUD can reduce hysterectomies, she wondered if *showing* them would work better.[93]

After reviewing the necessary literature, Dr. Phillips and a team of physicians went to work developing a toolkit of best practices for "diagnosing and treating benign conditions characterized by pelvic pain or uterine bleeding."[94] They turned to special effects specialists from the movie industry for help in creating a pelvic model, similar in size, shape and texture to a real woman. The model had to be as lifelike as possible for doctors to insert gel into the uterus, take tissue samples, fit pessaries (ring-like devices inserted into the vagina to support the organs following prolapse) and practise inserting the Mirena.

Once the prototype was fine-tuned into a final model, the researchers hit the road. They travelled across Ontario giving hands-on workshops for family physicians who wanted to learn some of these gynecological techniques. They even used a red, jam-like children's laxative to simulate uterine tissue so doctors could capture "tissue samples".

---

[93] Susan Phillips, "Does Hands-On CME in Gynaecologic Procedures Alter Clinical Practice?" *Medical Teacher* 32 (2010): 259-261.
[94] Susan Phillips, "Does Hands-On CME in Gynaecologic Procedures Alter Clinical Practice?," 259.

"We did a lot of thinking outside the box," says Dr. Risa Bordman, a family physician from Toronto and one of the researchers. "Obviously, education was a huge component as well. So we created an entire tool kit to help doctors diagnose the main benign conditions that lead to a hysterectomy. We produced a one-pager on each condition. The idea was just to try to get the physician or healthcare practitioner or nurse practitioner to make the proper diagnosis instead of sending every bleeding woman to a gynecologist."

The road show was such a success that Dr. Bordman, Dr. Phillips and the other researchers conducted "train the trainer" sessions and even took the pelvic model to medical schools. "Studies have shown that many women who have the Mirena IUD [for heavy menstrual bleeding] will not go ahead with a hysterectomy so it may be that family physicians and nurse practitioners hold the key to lowering hysterectomy rates," says Dr. Bordman.

The challenge in making that happen lies not so much in being able to prove the value of this kind of training, but rather in motivating physicians to attend such a workshop in the first place. "Once the physicians contemplate and accept the validity of an intervention, the participatory 'do more than one' approach evaluated in this study is an effective and satisfying method of delivering continuing medical education," concludes Dr. Phillips.[95]

Advantages

- This is a minimally invasive option that may lighten or stop your period for up to five years.

- It can be just as effective as surgery (endometrial ablation, to be discussed later) for bleeding.

---

[95] Susan Phillips, "Does Hands-On CME in Gynaecologic Procedures Alter Clinical Practice?," 261.

Disadvantages

- The Mirena doesn't work on everyone.

- As with any form of hormonal birth control, there can be side effects.

- There is a risk of uterine perforation.

An important safety note

In 2010, Health Canada, along with the Mirena manufacturer, Bayer, issued a bulletin to consumers regarding the potential risk of uterine perforation.[96] Bayer reported that it was receiving reports of perforation and that perforation occurs at a rate between 1 per 1,000 and 1 per 10,000 insertions. According to the company, the risk of perforation may be increased after pregnancy, during lactation and in women with unusual uterine anatomy.

---

[96] Health Canada, "Health Canada Endorsed Important Safety Information on MIRENA," www.hc-sc.gc.ca/dhp-mps/medeff/advisories-avis/prof/_2010/mirena_hpc-cps-eng.php (accessed June 2010).

Chapter 13

Hysteroscopy

A hysteroscopy is the procedure many gynecologists use to diagnose or treat certain conditions. A long, thin instrument called a hysteroscope is passed through the cervix and into the uterus to help the doctor find the cause of a problem or to confirm that your uterus is up to the challenge of surgery. Nowadays, these scopes have tiny cameras on the end of them so both you and your gynecologist can see the inside of your uterine cavity.

Hysteroscopies can be done in an outpatient clinic or in an operating room. Either way, you'll be given either a general or a regional anesthetic to block the pain or a sedative if you prefer to be awake. Depending on the type of procedure you're having, your doctor may also gently widen your cervix to allow the hysteroscope to enter your uterus more easily. Once the scope is inside, either gas or liquid is inserted through the scope to expand your uterus, making it easier to see the inside. If your doctor is trying to diagnose a problem, she will likely make a thorough examination and remove a tissue sample for further testing. If surgery is required, your doctor will insert small instruments through the hysteroscope to remove troublesome tissue such as polyps or fibroids. At the end of the procedure, the doctor removes the scope and the liquid and your uterus returns to normal.

Endometrial ablation

Another very common method of helping women lighten or stop their periods is endometrial ablation. Ablation can be effective for women who are finished having children or who don't wish to have children, but who would rather not undergo a hysterectomy.

The procedure preserves your uterus but not your ability to carry a child because the lining of your uterus, or endometrium, is cauterized during the procedure. Certain types of fibroids can also be destroyed during ablations, depending on their size and location.

Endometrial ablation has been used in Canada since the 1980s as a minimally invasive alternative to hysterectomy. There are two types of ablations – first and second generation. First-generation ablations are usually performed in hospital under local or regional anesthetic and require the surgeon to look directly inside the uterus through a hysteroscope while fluid is used to fill and expand the uterine cavity, giving the surgeon a wider view.

"The first-generation techniques offer considerable advantages over hysterectomy," says a report prepared for Santé Québec.[97] "They take less time to perform and require a much shorter hospital stay and convalescence. Although hysterectomy guarantees the cessation of menstrual flow and yields a higher level of satisfaction, it carries a greater risk of complications than endometrial ablation."

First-generation ablations

With this procedure, your doctor will first perform a hysteroscopy to check the integrity of your uterus and then proceed with the ablation.

The most common type of first-generation ablation is called a resectoscope, loop or rollerball ablation. Your doctor will use either a loop or small ball on the end of a scope to move around your uterus, like cutting a lawn, to physically cut out or burn the lining of the uterus. The rollerball or loop keeps going around and around until all the endometrial tissue is destroyed.

---

[97] Chantale Lessard and Alicia Framarin, *Endometrial Ablation Techniques in the Treatment of Dysfunctional Uterine Bleeding*, (Montreal: Agence d'évaluation des technologies et des modes d'intervention en santé Québec, 2002).

Advantages

- Minimally invasive

- Avoids a hysterectomy

- Can be done under local or regional anesthetic

- Tissue samples can be taken for biopsy

- Almost no pain after surgery

Disadvantages

- Requires a surgeon with experience

- Risk of uterine perforation

- Electrolyte (mineral) imbalance can be caused by too much fluid

Second-generation (thermal balloon) ablations

In this procedure, commonly known as a Thermablate or Thermachoice ablation, a small, soft, flexible balloon made of silicone is attached to a thin catheter (tube) and passed through the vagina and cervix and into the uterus. The balloon is then filled with fluid so that it inflates to the contours of the uterus. The fluid is then heated and circulated in the uterus for eight minutes while the lining of the uterus is destroyed. When the treatment is completed, the fluid is taken out of the balloon and the catheter is removed.

 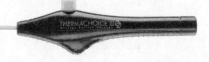

A device used to perform a thermal balloon ablation.

Advantages

- Minimally invasive

- Avoids a hysterectomy

- Can be done under local or regional anesthetic

- Fast

Disadvantages

- Can be done only on certain size and shape uteruses

- Length of surgery can vary

Second-generation (bipolar mesh) ablations

The bipolar mesh ablation, more commonly known by its trade name, NovaSure, is a second-generation ablation that is growing in popularity among many Canadian gynecologists.

"Although ablations such as [first-generation] resectoscopic ablations are just as effective as [bipolar mesh] ablations, the risks of resectoscopic ablations are higher," says Dr. Singh. "The fluid used to distend the uterine cavity may lead to fluid overload and/or an electrolyte imbalance, which can be life-threatening. There is also greater skill required for the resectoscopic approach and perforation of the uterus or bleeding may occur. These newer procedures are more user-friendly and require less time without the need to distend the cavity with fluid."

How they work

Bipolar mesh ablations can be done either in an office-type outpatient clinic (there are only a handful of these in Canada) or in an operating room. With an office-based ablation, the patient is given a mild sedative for relaxation and a bit of local anesthetic through the cervix. She lies back on a reclining dentist-type

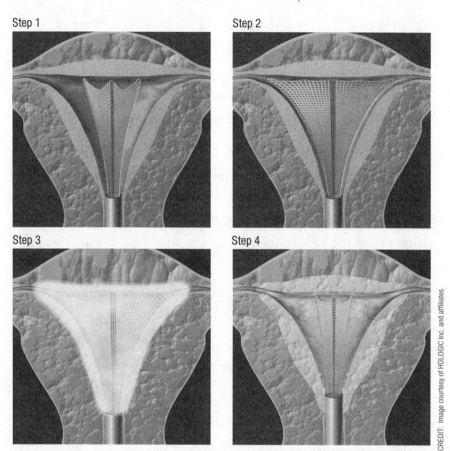

Step 1

Step 2

Step 3

Step 4

CREDIT: Image courtesy of HOLOGIC Inc. and affiliates.

NovaSure endometrial ablation system. Step 1: A slender wand is inserted into the uterus. Step 2: A mesh emerges from the wand. Step 3: The mesh expands to the contours of the uterus and begins ablating the endometrium. Step 4: The mesh is retracted and the device is removed from the uterus.

chair with her feet in stirrups. The gynecologist then inserts a hysteroscope through the cervix and into the uterus to check the size, shape and condition of the uterine cavity. A live picture of the cavity is projected on a plasma screen through a tiny camera located on the tip of the hysteroscope.

The hysteroscope is then removed from the uterus and a slender wand, which is connected to a nearby computer, is inserted into the uterine cavity. A mesh emerges from the wand and gently expands to the exact size and shape of the uterus through input it receives from the computer. Then, precisely measured radio frequency energy is delivered through the mesh for about 90 seconds, coagulating (destroying) the lining of the uterus. The mesh device is then pulled back into the wand and both are removed from the uterus.

The entire procedure takes about five minutes, after which the patient goes to a recovery room for about an hour before going home. The procedure would be almost exactly the same in an operating room, but the woman may be put under general anesthetic.

The Shirley E. Greenberg Women's Health Centre in Ottawa is one of the few centres in Canada that offers bipolar mesh ablations in an outpatient setting. I took a tour of the minimally invasive outpatient suite there and have posted a video on my website (unhysterectomy.com).

Advantages

- It's minimally invasive.

- It can be used even if you have small fibroids and polyps.

- It can be done in an outpatient setting with sedation or in an operating room under full anesthetic.

- It's fast.

- You can return to your normal activities the same day.

Disadvantages

- You may have a bit of cramping and spotting after the procedure.

- There is risk of infection, uterine perforation or thermal injury (these risks are lower than with first-generation techniques).

- It does not preserve fertility.

Why everyone isn't having one

But only in Canada could something so sensible be so political. You would think that with the number of women having hysterectomies in Canada, and the number who are so desperate to find less-invasive solutions, women would be beating a path to the nearest hospital to demand these types of ablations. Sadly, they're not. I daresay most Canadian women are unaware the procedure even exists. Brenda is a perfect example. Even as a nurse who bled profusely for many years, Brenda became aware of bipolar mesh ablations only after she started assisting gynecologists with performing them in the Women's Health Centre at the Regina General Hospital.

"It was amazing," she says. "I spent so many years bleeding, thinking it was normal and just something I had to put up with and then I started seeing all these women coming in for these ablations and literally walking out the door an hour later and going back to work. I thought 'Hey, this is for me,' so I went to my doctor and asked for a referral and I got it done."

Brenda went home that night, and despite some cramping and a bit of spotting, she was back to her normal routine in a few hours. She has not had a period since, saying her bleeding is 99.9 percent better.

Under our current healthcare system, however, bipolar mesh ablations are very hard to come by. Even though the procedure has the potential to radically alter the way we treat HMB in this country, and reduce the number of unnecessary hysterectomies significantly, it's simply not happening as often as it should be. In Ontario, for example, the devices used to perform ablations, which cost about $1,000 each, are not covered by the Ontario Health Insurance Plan so hospitals must pay for them (if they decide to offer them at all) out of their global operating budgets, the budgets they receive from their provincial health ministries. As a result, many hospitals in Ontario and in other provinces cap the number of bipolar mesh ablations they will do every year. Once their yearly quotas are filled, hospitals stop offering them, leaving women to bleed. The women either go back on the waiting list for NovaSure ablations the following year, or for more invasive surgery such as a hysterectomy.

Unfortunately, under global operating budgets, hospitals have only so much money to go around. Everyone is clamouring for a piece of the pie – gynecologists, internists, orthopedic surgeons, oncologists, you name it. Hospital administrators are in a no-win situation. With their provincial masters breathing down their necks to reduce wait times for higher-priority surgeries for things like cancer and joint replacements, hospitals must borrow from Peter to pay Paul, or not borrow anything at all. Cancer will always trump HMB, and so it should.

What I have a problem with is the fact that such a competition exists in the first place. There should be enough money to go around for all of us, and there could be if our politicians and healthcare policy-makers would think outside the box long enough to see the logic in taking these five-minute ablations out of expensive operating rooms and putting them into community outpatient clinics or ambulatory clinics in hospitals. In doing so, we could save millions, if not billions, of dollars in the long run, treat more women and free up our precious operating rooms for those who really need them, such as cancer patients. The whole system is upside down.

Dr. Leyland explains how the current funding formula plays out in his hospital every day. "New technologies, to be embraced within the system, have to be taken out of other resources. So in other words, a hospital administrator would come to me and say, 'Dr. Leyland, what are you *not* going to do next year so that you can provide this particular type of new technology this year?' And unfortunately, that's the reality that we're facing. It is very frustrating because we know that there are standards of care now that we're developing that are much better for women, where they can come and have a procedure done and go back to their activities of daily living much faster than having a hysterectomy or other major intervention – back to their families, back to their work. It's certainly better economically for society. But we're limited in how many of these procedures we can perform, or in even being *able* to offer the procedures."

Dr. Hassan Shenassa, a gynecologist in Ottawa at the Shirley E. Greenberg Women's Health Centre who performs outpatient NovaSure ablations, explains the situation from the hospital's point of view. "If we replace hysterectomy cases with office-based ablations [still inside a hospital, just not in an operating room], the devices must still be paid for so unless I close the operating room, I'm not actually saving the hospital any money. The operating room is still filled with other cases because the need is there. So in actual fact we are *adding* extra costs and never really saving the hospital any money. I appreciate that it's a concern, but we just have to look at healthcare differently in Canada."

Dr. Andrew Browning, a gynecologist at the Royal Victoria Hospital in Barrie, Ontario, found a rather novel way to convince his hospital administrators to remove the yearly quotas on bipolar mesh ablations: he simply asked them to.

> The bottom line is it was pretty clear that thermal ablation was becoming the standard of care for menorrhagia and it just seemed like it was a difficult situation if there was a cap to try to determine who would get this type of a procedure and who wouldn't. It would be an unfair situation, and hence the combination of being able to explain to our administration the importance of being able to offer the procedure and the inability to differentiate who should get it and who shouldn't, led our administration to realize that it certainly is an important procedure that we should be offering in this community.

> If you look at hospitals in Ontario right now that don't offer a procedure like NovaSure, I think it's really astounding in the sense that there's no doubt in my mind, or in anybody's who does these, that it's an incredible procedure that is profoundly successful 97 percent of the time. The fact that you can offer someone that procedure and it only takes about five minutes with a very low complication rate means that it's really something that should be offered to anyone who wants it in Ontario, in my opinion. The only reason not to be able to offer it is a financial decision on the part of a hospital and I think that's something worth our time as gynecologists – to advocate for our patients that a procedure like this really should be offered throughout Ontario.

Whether it's Ontario, Alberta or Newfoundland, one could say the issue is one of philosophy. How important are quality of life procedures for women compared with life-saving surgery for cancer or heart and lung disease? Under global operating budgets, hospitals must constantly weigh which procedures are *more important* than others. But the situation isn't entirely grim; in Manitoba, for example, women from northern areas such as Rankin Inlet or Hudson's Bay are routinely flown down to Winnipeg to have the procedure done.

Dr. Leyland believes the solution is to establish freestanding provincially funded outpatient clinics, known as Independent

Health Facilities, similar to ones set up for bariatric surgery. "These ablations cost between $1,000 and $2,000. On the other hand, hysterectomies, on average, not including costs to the family, time off work and the economic impact on society, cost somewhere between $3,000 and $4,000. So obviously, there are very effective ways of providing this kind of care by just shifting resources around.

"I believe this is a common-sense solution, but the unfortunate thing is that our healthcare system is very much hospital-centric, so we need to have a complete paradigm shift in how we can provide this kind of care. And that kind of change is extremely difficult to implement within the Canadian healthcare system because it's also very, very politicized."

Dr. Leyland says gynecologists have been asking for these independent health facilities for years, to no avail. Perhaps it's time for us, as women, to lend our voices to their plea. "Politicians respond to political pressure," Dr. Leyland says, "and political pressure doesn't come from the Ontario Medical Association or the physicians. It really has to come from patients, because they're the legitimate owners of our healthcare system."

If you feel as strongly as I do that this situation has to change, please contact your local hospital to find out if they impose quotas on procedures such as bipolar mesh ablations, or write to your provincial minister of health or local member of provincial parliament to request that hospitals remove quotas on ablations immediately. If we turn up the volume on this issue, our politicians will indeed have to listen.

Are ablations more cost-effective than hysterectomies?

A study in 1996 by the Department of Obstetrics and Gynecology at St. Joseph's Health Centre at the University of

Western Ontario in London found ablations to be 82 percent more effective and 58 percent less expensive (in terms of overall cost) than vaginal hysterectomies for the treatment of women with HMB.[98]

The total cost for each procedure was about $5,273 per vaginal hysterectomy and $2,279 per hysteroscopic endometrial ablation, a saving of $3,094.

The study also found that vaginal hysterectomy eliminated bleeding in 100 percent of patients and had a complication rate of 41 percent. Endometrial ablation eliminated or improved bleeding in 90 percent of patients (amenorrhea, or no periods, 46 percent; hypomenorrhea [short or scanty periods], 35 percent; eumenorrhea [normal menstruation], nine percent; no significant change, 10 percent). No complications were associated with ablation and it resulted in 82 percent patient satisfaction.

Many studies have compared the efficacy and cost-effectiveness of minimally invasive surgery, intrauterine devices, medications and hysterectomy. My goal is not to provide the definitive comparison between approaches, but rather to offer a glimpse into what experts in minimally invasive gynecology have studied. In the University of Western Ontario study, the authors are some of the most highly respected gynecologists in the world and I believe we should, at a minimum, take their findings into consideration. I realize times have changed since 1996, especially where healthcare costs are concerned, but I can assure you the main philosophy behind minimally invasive gynecology has not changed since then: it's simply better for the patient.

---

[98] G.A. Vilos, J.T Pispidikis and C.K. Botz, "Economic Evaluation of Hysteroscopic Endometrial Ablation versus Vaginal Hysterectomy for Menorrhagia," *Obstetrics and Gynecology* 88, no. 2 (Aug. 1996): 241-5.

Chapter 14
Focused Ultrasound, Uterine Artery Embolization
and Volumetric Embolization

The next procedures I'm going to discuss bring a whole new meaning to the words *minimally invasive* surgery; in fact, you might even say they are *non-invasive*, or completely scarless. Unlike traditional surgery, which requires large incisions using instruments such as scalpels, or even minimally invasive surgery, which employs fewer, smaller incisions and uses scopes, focused ultrasound and uterine artery embolization require *no* incisions.

Focused ultrasound

Focused ultrasound is nothing new. As far back as the 1950s, researchers investigated its potential as a replacement for invasive surgery. Unfortunately, at the time of those early experiments, there was no imaging system to allow doctors to "see" their targets (mostly tumours) and no way to provide heated imaging. Heated, or thermal, imaging uses ultrasound energy to raise the temperature of the targeted tissue and cause the tissue to coagulate.

Today, however, technology exists that allows physicians to use focused ultrasound energy to target tissue located deep inside the body to achieve a specific, therapeutic result. In the case of fibroids, focused ultrasound can literally zap the tumours completely non-invasively. When combined with magnetic resonance imaging (MRI) – which allows physicians to target specific tissue and receive instant feedback about whether the therapy was successful – focused ultrasound puts medicine on the brink of revolutionizing the way we treat illness.

Although magnetic resonance-guided focused ultrasound surgery (MRgFUS) is exciting for its possible use in treating fibroids, researchers are examining ways of using it to treat a number of conditions, including brain tumours. Often referred to as a "scarless" procedure, MRgFUS uses focused, or targeted, ultrasound waves to heat and destroy fibroids using high-frequency, high-energy sound waves without affecting any nearby tissue or organs. MRgFUS treatment for fibroids takes about three hours and is an attractive treatment option for women with HMB because it stops your bleeding while sparing your uterus.

Fifty-six-year-old Ruth from northwest England contacted me through Facebook to explain why she went looking for focused ultrasound in her country. And just like Canadian and American women I have heard from, Ruth encountered problems accessing the procedure:

> I'm a bit of a freak of nature as I'm 56 and appear to be nowhere near menopause. What I thought was a combination of menopause and aging for the last couple of years turned out to be fibroids. I have heavy bleeding and bloating and I can't leave the house for several days when it's at its worst. Plus the pressure on my bladder is very uncomfortable. I'm only seven stone, 10 pounds (108 pounds) and I look five months pregnant.

> I was diagnosed with fibroids last August, one at nearly six centimetres and two smaller ones between two and three centimetres. My uterus is the size of a 16–20 week pregnancy. My GP offered me a Mirena IUD or a hysterectomy. The Mirena would help the bleeding but wouldn't reduce the size of the fibroids, plus [the doctor said it would be] difficult to insert in a uterus with fibroids and there was a risk of perforation and infection. I already knew there were other options but my GP said they weren't available in my area. I asked to be referred to someone else and she agreed so off I went to find out more.

> To make a long story short, I decided focused ultrasound was the very best option. It's pain-free, non-invasive and the recovery time is one day. It's a no brainer. I managed to find the only hospital in the UK that does

it and the only professor who does the procedure under the National Health Service. I emailed her and was accepted as a patient. I had an MRI last September which showed I was suitable for treatment. I went to her clinic in December, where she decided to fast track me and started the funding bid the same day. (In the UK, it is the Primary Care Trust [PCT] that decides whether or not to fund treatment outside of a patient's area). The funding was rejected in February 2012 based on cost (which was confusing since focused ultrasound is cheaper than hysterectomy), lack of long-term outcome (because of my age I was considered irrelevant, I guess) and equity (why should I be given treatment that is unavailable to other women). My reply was "Why shouldn't I be given treatment which other women's PCT's are funding."

It has been a long road to get this far but I am completely at peace that it is the right thing to do, grateful that my condition isn't life-threatening so I don't have to rush into any decisions and absolutely thrilled to have the most powerful woman in her field fighting in my corner for me.

I am not militantly "anti-hysterectomy." I just don't think it should be done routinely for conditions that aren't life-threatening. I'd rather let nature take its course at my age. All I want is a bridge to natural menopause and if you could invent a treatment for that it would be focused ultrasound.

I have access to medical databases as part of my job and I did my level best to find "cons" as well as "pros" for this treatment and really there are scarcely any. From what I could find, the worst-case scenario is that the fibroids can grow back, as they can with any treatment apart from hysterectomy. But at my age I don't think they'll have time to and that is the basis of the appeal.

So long as I don't look five months gone at my daughter's wedding in October, or bleed through my bride's mother's dress, I'll be happy.

At the time of writing, Ruth had submitted her appeal and was waiting for a date to appear before the appeal panel. Watch my website for updates on her health and her appeal.

Focused ultrasound in Canada

Although focused ultrasound is available in the UK, and has been used in the US since 2000 under the brand name ExAblate, the procedure is not yet available in Canada; however, clinical trials of MRgFUS are underway in Ontario. In 2010, the Thunder Bay Regional Health Sciences Centre and Sunnybrook Health Sciences Centre in Toronto partnered to create a unique dual-centred site to investigate treatments for various conditions using MRgFUS. Interestingly, researchers chose fibroids as the subject of their first investigations. Early results from the trials are promising. The treatment is said to be "safe and effective with no serious side effects."

Dr. Kullervo Hynynen, a professor in the Department of Medical Biophysics at the University of Toronto and the director of imaging at Sunnybrook, is a pioneer of MRgFUS technology. He's also a co-investigator on the fibroid trials in Toronto, which are being led by Dr. Elizabeth David, an interventional radiologist at Sunnybrook. Dr. Laura Curiel is leading the research at Thunder Bay Regional Research Institute with clinical leads Dr. Neety Panu, a radiologist at the Linda Buchan Centre, Thunder Bay Regional Health Sciences Centre, and Dr. Andrew Siren, obstetrician and gynecologist at the Thunder Bay Regional Health Sciences Centre.

"These clinical trials are significant both in future treatment availability in Canada, and in informing our imminent work on non-invasive treatments for cancer patients as well," says Dr. Hynynen. The researchers plan to expand trials for the treatment of various types of tumours.

During the procedure, patients lie inside the MRI scanner, which produces three-dimensional images of the problematic tissue. This allows physicians to direct precise, high-intensity, focused ultrasound waves into the body at specific targets – the problematic tissue – at temperatures of between 65° and 85°C, destroying the tissue. Owing to the thermal imaging provided by the MRI scanner, physicians get real-time feedback on how well the procedure is progressing, which gives them tremendous control over the outcome of the procedure. Each pulse lasts about 15 seconds and is repeated about 50 times throughout the procedure.

"This particular type of treatment is just an ultrasound beam that's focused so there's absolutely no incision, no scarring and very little post-operative care," says Dr. David. "It's truly non-invasive."

Advantages

- This is a non-invasive treatment employing no incisions and leaving no scars.

- Women can return home after the treatment and are back to their normal activities within two to three days.

Disadvantages

- It may be uncomfortable for some women to lie on their stomach for the three hours it takes to perform the procedure. Pain medication and sedatives can be given.

- This procedure is designed for women who have completed their childbearing or don't intend to have children.

- It is still too early to say whether MRgFUS provides long-term relief from symptoms.

Watch my website for updates on the Canadian MRgFUS trials.

Uterine artery embolization

Uterine artery embolization (UAE) is another exciting minimally invasive treatment option for uterine fibroids. The first report on UAE was published in the medical journal *The Lancet*[99] in 1995; it is a widely accepted form of treatment for shrinking fibroids while preserving the reproductive organs. It has yet to be

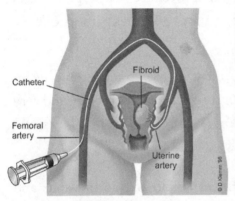

The uterine artery embolization procedure.

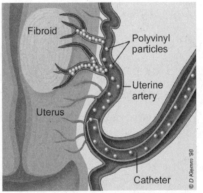

Microspheres, or polyvinyl particles, being delivered during uterine artery embolization.

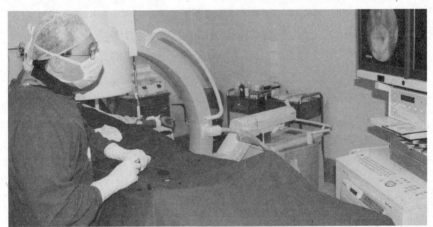

Uterine artery embolization being performed on a patient.

---

[99] www.lancet.com

proven, however, whether UAE affects fertility. More research is needed in this area. Unlike MRgFUS, UAE typically takes only an hour and does not involve lying on your stomach.

How uterine artery embolization works

With UAE, patients are taken to the angiography, or medical imaging, suite and are placed on a special table. The procedure is done with the patient lying on her back. The physician, an interventional radiologist, makes a tiny nick in your groin to allow access to the femoral artery in your upper thigh.

The radiologist then uses special x-ray equipment to guide a catheter (a small tube) from the femoral artery to the uterine artery. When the uterine artery is reached, small plastic particles, called microspheres, are delivered through the catheter into the blood that leads to the uterus. The interventional radiologist then moves the catheter to the uterine artery on the other side of the uterus and injects more particles. The particles block the vessels around the fibroid, choking off the oxygen supply that fibroids need in order to grow. The oxygen deprivation makes the fibroids shrink. The microspheres stay in the blood vessels permanently. Once the embolization is complete, the catheter is removed and the physician applies pressure on the nick to stop it from bleeding.

Hope Waltman, an outspoken American IT professional-turned- uterine fibroid patient advocate, had the UAE procedure in September 2001 after discovering she had fibroids during an annual routine visit to her gynecologist. She was not impressed with his approach.

He said to me, "Oh, by the way, did we ever discuss your fibroids that are growing?" I looked at him really dumb, like, "What is he talking about?" My first thought at the moment was, How long had I had these things and why didn't he let me know before? He put me on a prescription pain killer but the discomfort got so bad that even that didn't take the pain away. I was miserable. I mean, I would just be walking the floor. If I was at work I would just sit there and be holding onto the desk. I didn't want to tell anybody that I was in pain, but I was.

It just made me mad because my gynecologist immediately started talking about surgery (hysterectomy or myomectomy) and he never once brought up uterine artery embolization or any other options. Even though I had seen my gynecologist for 15 years, I ended up finding another gynecologist away from my area in Philly. This gyn explained to my husband and me every option in great detail and even gave me some brochures to take home. I told [the new doctor] I was thinking of UAE and going to an interventional radiologist and he told me there was no reason why I couldn't have the procedure.

When I had the procedure done, antibiotics were administered and choices of conscious sedation or spinal analgesia were offered. Some women will become so relaxed that they will fall asleep during the procedure. I talked to the interventional radiologist and watched him while he performed the procedure and I saw the x-ray screen he was using to see my arteries. I was able to experience the whole thing.

Hope experienced a bit of cramping (similar to menstrual cramps) after the procedure from the loss of blood supply to the fibroids. She managed the cramps using a patient-controlled analgesia pump, which usually uses morphine and later over-the-counter pain medications and some prescription medicine. About 90 percent of patients go home the same day. It took about three months for the fibroids to shrink and approximately three to six months more for Hope's uterus to return to its normal size, but after that, her periods became lighter, her ovulation pain was gone and she entered menopause naturally.

"I think somebody from above was kind of there for us," she said, "because my husband and I had such doubts in our minds from what the previous gynecologist had suggested, and that prompted us to go looking for more information. I was glad that both my husband and I had the feeling that we needed to do this."

Which is better, UAE or MRgFUS?

The Center for Uterine Fibroids at the Mayo Clinic in Rochester, Minnesota, and Duke University at Durham, North Carolina, are conducting the first study[100] to compare uterine artery embolization and magnetic resonance-guided focused ultrasound surgery for the treatment of fibroids. The study, called Fibroid Interventions: Reducing Symptoms Today and Tomorrow (FIRSTT), will follow women for three years to assess how effective the treatments are in terms of symptom relief, side effects, impact on quality of life, need for additional treatment and even the costs associated with each approach.

The primary goal of the study is to compare the safety and effectiveness of these two standard fibroid treatments. A second goal is to better understand which symptoms bother women with fibroids the most, in order to find the best possible treatment outcomes for women and to control healthcare costs.

Dr. Elizabeth Stewart is the lead investigator of the study. We're actually doing what you call a randomized clinical trial, which is considered the gold standard. So a couple of years down the road, we'll be able to tell if one treatment is absolutely better than the other, or if one treatment is better for women who have this kind of fibroid or this kind of complaint, and really to be able to answer some of the important questions in the field."

---

[100] E.V. Bouwsma, G.K. Hesley, D.A. Woodrum, A.L. Weaver, P.C. Leppert, L.G. Peterson and E.A. Stewart, "Comparing Focused Ultrasound and Uterine Artery Embolization for Uterine Fibroids-Rationale and Design of the Fibroid Interventions: Reducing Symptoms Today and Tomorrow (FIRSTT) Trial," *Fertility and Sterility* 96 no. 3 (Sept. 2011): 704-10

Although this study, and the one in Toronto and Thunder Bay, is extremely promising, science still has a long way to go in getting to the root of what causes HMB in the first place. Dr. Stewart explains how countries such as Canada and the US can encourage further investigation.

I think it takes three things. It takes physicians and scientists who are willing to do the work; it takes a funding mechanism, because these are not seen as high-priority issues so it's often hard to get funding from governments or foundations or bodies like that. But I think it also takes women who are willing to enrol in the studies and that's a really hard thing to do. Women who are suffering may say, "I'm not going to make the decision about what treatment I'm going to get until I look at my options" and that may prolong her suffering.

And so I think that's why we're excited about [studying] focused ultrasound and uterine artery embolization, because I believe they're both good choices compared to hysterectomy for many women. And you know, many women do feel comfortable with that option, especially when they say, "Gee, you know, if this is going to help my daughter, who may have the same problem in 10 or 20 years," then that's a reasonable thing to do, and women all over will benefit from this information.

We've spent so much of our time focusing on doing hysterectomies that we haven't studied the biology of fibroids. So there are likely even more alternatives to hysterectomy out there, and hopefully even ways to prevent them, that will be understood within the next decade. I like to use the analogy of what happened in the 1960s around heart disease. There was a push to establish coronary care units to better take care of people with heart attacks. And I think we're there now with fibroids. We have focused ultrasound. We have uterine artery embolization. We have minimally invasive options. But with heart disease they went further and asked, "What actually causes heart disease?" And then they established that high cholesterol is linked to heart disease so they began to treat high cholesterol and so on and so forth.

So I think that yes, we have a problem with women not hearing about all of the good options, but the even bigger problem is that we haven't invested money in research to find out more about the disease itself in order to create better options.

Whether you choose UAE, MRgFUS or any of the other options discussed in this book, the take-away message is this: you have options. After everything she experienced, Hope Waltman has a very strong message for women about the issue of choice.

> When a woman/patient is first diagnosed with fibroids, the first thing that pops into her mind is that something, "a tumour," is growing inside of my uterus/body. Needless to say it can be a frightening moment and it is hard to concentrate on what the doctor is telling you. Don't panic.

> I highly recommend that you take a friend/partner with you to the examination/consultation so that you have someone who asks questions and listens to what the doctor says to you. If the doctor doesn't take time to explain to you all the fibroid procedures, it may be a good idea to get a second or third doctor's opinion (gynecologist and interventional radiologist) before making a decision. Remember, not every doctor is the same. The doctors may have the same MD after their name, but that doesn't mean they know or have the same skill or expertise in every procedure, medical device, etc. Ask the doctor what procedures he or she performs, their training record, how many procedures they've performed, pros and cons of each procedure, maintaining fertility for a future family, surgical menopause and success rates.

> With all the procedures that are out there women have more options today than ever before and hysterectomy should not be the first one on the list unless cancer or another medical problem is a concern, or the woman (not just the doctor) decides she wants the hysterectomy. Women should remember, it is your body!

For more information you can contact Hope Waltman. Her website is hopeforfibroids.org and her email address is hope@hopeforfibroids.org.

If you are an American, you can find out more about enrolling in the FIRSTT study by contacting Lisa G. Peterson, RN, at 507-266-4813 or by email at mayofibroids@mayo.edu. Watch my website for updates on both studies as they become available.

Volumetric ablation

A new type of fibroid ablation device called the VizAblate system is approved for use in Europe and is also being further studied in the European Union and Mexico. VizAblate uses radiofrequency energy to perform what is called "volumetric ablation" in which the volume of the fibroid that is heated and destroyed is tailored to the volume of the fibroid itself.

With this type of ablation system, the physician places a device through the cervix into the uterus. From within the uterus, the physician can see and selectively target each fibroid using a handpiece that has both ultrasound and radiofrequency electrodes, which are controlled by computer software. The electrodes are then inserted into the fibroid and radiofrequency energy is used to heat, or ablate, the fibroid. After the ablation is over, the handpiece is removed. The procedure is performed without incisions and patients can return home within a few hours.

"Instead of making a series of blind ablations into a fibroid multiple times, we can make one ablation that has been sized to that specific fibroid," says Dr. David Toub, medical director of Gynesonics, the company that developed the VizAblate system.

This device is a first because we've married radiofrequency ablation for treatment with intrauterine ultrasound for imaging into one device. So while radiofrequency energy is fairly established, intrauterine ultrasound is fairly new. It's really only used with our device. And it allows us to see far more than we can see with hysteroscopy within the uterus. We can see the myometrium (the middle layer of the uterine wall), we can see the uterine serosa (membrane), we can even see some things outside the uterus such as the ovaries and bowel. Radiofrequency ablation has been around a long time and ultrasound has been around a long time but it's hard to do. You have a device in one hand and an ultrasound in the other so it can be cumbersome. By putting this all on one device, I think that's much more usable.

A lot of us in laparoscopy and hysteroscopy are very visual people. We need to see what we're doing. So the ultrasound allows us to see where the ablation will take place and where the heat will go. You can essentially plan your ablation before you ever put any electrodes into the fibroid. There are no incisions, no laparoscopy but we do need some degree of anesthesia, although this even potentially can be an office procedure. We've done this under conscious sedation with very good results. And I'm delighted that we have a group of physicians in the European Union and in Mexico who are using this device, certainly with our trial.

Volumetric ablation is not approved for use in Canada or the US and there is no conclusive evidence yet on its effect on fertility.

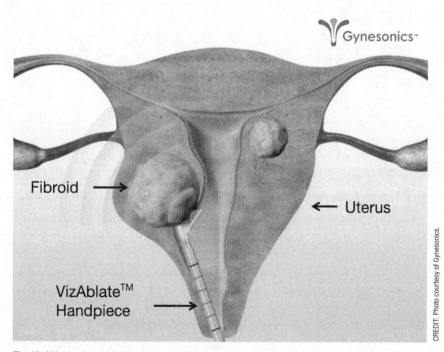

The VizAblate volumetric ablation system.

Chapter 15
Myomectomy

The word myomectomy stems from the words leiomyoma or myoma, both of which mean fibroid. The term used to describe the surgery to remove a myoma is myomectomy. As with hysterectomies, there are three ways to perform a myomectomy: hysteroscopically, laparoscopically and abdominally.

Methods
Hysteroscopic

Myomectomy can be done hysteroscopically, or vaginally, through a lit hysteroscope with a camera that is passed through the cervix into the uterus. This method is used to remove fibroids on the inner wall of the uterus that have not grown deep into the uterine wall. Hysteroscopic myomectomy can be done as outpatient surgery, without a general anesthetic if the patient prefers, requires no overnight stay and recovery is one day to two weeks. Hysteroscopic myomectomy is considered the least invasive, most conservative approach to removing fibroids while sparing the uterus.[101]

Laparoscopic

Laparoscopic myomectomy is performed through three or four small incisions (usually all less than a centimetre) in the abdomen. This requires surgical skills not widely available, but it offers greater ability to remove larger fibroids that cannot be removed with the hysteroscopic approach. Recovery is much quicker than with a laparotomy (larger incision) and it may result in less scarring inside the abdomen.

---

[101] Grace Liu, Lynne Zolis, Rose Kung, Mary Melchior, Sukhbir Singh and Francis Cook, "The Laparoscopic Myomectomy: A Survey of Canadian Gynecologists," *Journal of Obstetrics and Gynaecology Canada*, 32 (Feb. 2010).

Abdominal

Abdominal myomectomy is done through a bikini or midline incision along the abdomen. This method is usually used to remove large or multiple fibroids or fibroids that have grown deep into the uterine wall. Abdominal myomectomy requires a two- to four-night stay in hospital and recovery time is between four and six weeks. This is the way most myomectomies are done in North America.

Advantages

- Minimally invasive if done laparoscopically or vaginally
- Removes only the fibroids, not the reproductive organs
- Preserves fertility

Disadvantages

- Fibroids can return
- Scar tissue may form
- If done abdominally, recovery can be long

Why are myomectomies done?

Myomectomy is the preferred surgery for women who want to preserve their fertility or who are past childbearing but want to avoid a hysterectomy. Here are three other common reasons for choosing this approach:

- To treat anemia that is not relieved through medication
- To relieve pain, pressure and HMB caused by fibroids
- To improve the chances of pregnancy in a woman whose fibroids have changed the wall of the uterus, which can sometimes cause infertility or miscarriages; myomectomies are sometimes done before in vitro fertilization is attempted

The procedure has two phases. Phase one begins about three to six months before surgery with gonadotropin-releasing hormone analogue (GnRH-a) therapy. Your gynecologist will put you into medically induced menopause to make your fibroids smaller and easier to remove during surgery. GnRH-a therapy may also reduce your risk of blood loss. Phase two is the surgery itself.

Accessibility

Like hysterectomies, the majority of myomectomies are still being done abdominally, when they're done at all. Some gynecologists are simply reluctant to perform myomectomies because of the risk of blood loss.

A survey[102] of 1,279 obstetrician-gynecologists on the Society of Obstetricians and Gynecologists of Canada mailing list released in the February 2010 issue of the *Journal of Obstetrics and Gynaecology Canada* produced the following results:

- Of the 529 obstetrician-gynecologists who responded to the survey, 24.5 percent performed laparoscopic myomectomy, but only 3.1 percent stated that more than half of their myomectomies were performed laparoscopically.

- 212 gynecologists (44.3 percent) said they had referred a patient to another gynecologist for a laparoscopic myomectomy.

- Laparoscopic surgeons felt the principal barrier to performing laparoscopic myomectomy was lack of training in the procedure.

---

[102] Grace Liu, Lynne Zolis, Rose Kung, Mary Melchior, Sukhbir Singh and Francis Cook, "The Laparoscopic Myomectomy: A Survey of Canadian Gynecologists," *Journal of Obstetrics and Gynaecology Canada*.

- 70.7 percent of the gynecologists felt the principal barrier to referring patients to another gynecologist for laparoscopic myomectomy was *their uncertainty about who offered the procedure.*

- The majority of respondents were unsure which procedure is superior with respect to blood loss, scar formation, postprocedure fertility rate, uterine rupture rate in subsequent pregnancy and cost-effectiveness.[103]

Dr. Wolfman says,

After the decision has been made to operate, there are several considerations when deciding the best surgical approach for fibroids. (Usually this occurs after a trial of conservative or medical therapy and a discussion of techniques such as embolization.)

1. The patient's anatomy may not be conducive to a minimalistic approach. The uterus may be too large or there may be too many fibroids to do a minimalistic approach. Only certain fibroids that are located inside the uterine cavity can be removed via a hysteroscope.

2. The patient has completed her childbearing. Myomectomy can be a bloody operation. Complications include the possibility of a blood transfusion, adhesion formation to the bowel, bladder or other structures, which may cause pain. Ultimately a hysterectomy may have to be done. Reoccurrence of fibroids is a possibility. Rarely (in about one percent of cases or less) the fibroids may be malignant. For all these reasons, most gynecologists recommend a total or sub-total hysterectomy when a woman is finished her childbearing. Exceptions might include the removal of a single large fibroid or fibroids located inside the uterus.

3. There may be other gynecologic diseases in the pelvis, such as ovarian cysts or endometriosis. A laparoscopic approach may still be possible in these situations.

4. The surgeon is not trained in minimalistic laparoscopic techniques.

5. The patient has other medical problems that preclude a minimalistic approach.

---

[103] Grace Liu, Lynne Zolis, Rose Kung, Mary Melchior, Sukhbir Singh and Francis Cook, "The Laparoscopic Myomectomy: A Survey of Canadian Gynecologists," *Journal of Obstetrics and Gynaecology Canada*, 147.

Each situation is different and the decision is made based on the patient's medical history, anatomy and wishes, and the equipment available to the surgeon in the operating room.

The American experience

Laparoscopic myomectomies, and hysterectomies for that matter, seem to have been around a lot longer in the US than in Canada. Dr. Parker, author of *A Gynecologist's Second Opinion*, has been performing laparoscopic myomectomies for 20 years.

Laparoscopic surgery differs from traditional surgery in a few key ways: during laparoscopic surgery, the surgeon is not looking into the abdomen directly through a large incision across the abdomen, but performs the surgery while looking at a large video monitor suspended over the patient's abdomen. The surgery, and especially the suturing of the uterus that is necessary during a laparoscopic myomectomy, requires a great deal of hand-eye coordination and dexterity, as well as knowledge of pelvic anatomy, in order to be successful.

The procedure is very safe and effective when performed by a properly trained physician and the technique continues to evolve as new instruments are developed. However, many physicians today still lack the skills necessary to perform myomectomies through the laparoscope and therefore do not offer them to patients. Because of the small size of the incisions and the level of skill needed to correctly perform the surgery, this procedure is actually harder for a physician to perform without the proper experience and takes more skill and training than abdominal surgery.

I began performing operative laparoscopic procedures in 1987 and have been performing laparoscopic myomectomies for nearly 20 years. I have been teaching these techniques to other gynecologists since 1990 and am an internationally recognized expert in fibroid surgery and research. I am considered one of the best fibroid surgeons for laparoscopic or abdominal myomectomy in the United States and abroad and am able to perform laparoscopic myomectomy surgery with minimal blood loss, a short time under anesthesia for the patient and with consistently good outcomes.[104]

---

[104] William Parker, "What Is a Laparoscopic Myomectomy?" 2012. www.fibroidsecondopinion.com/myomectomy.

To Canadians, that may sound like an advertisement – and it is. American physicians are paid by their patients, or their patients' insurance companies, not through publically funded healthcare, so who can blame them for selling their wares? Canadian doctors are forbidden by law to advertise, which makes it extremely difficult for patients to find specialists who can perform minimally invasive surgery. (See Chapter 18 to meet a Canadian woman who spent $25,000 of her own money to have a laparoscopic myomectomy in the United States.)

Myomectomy from the patients' perspective

For women like me, who are past childbearing, a myomectomy holds the promise of relief without having to surrender our uterus for whatever reason, be it sentimental, physical or otherwise. Gail Thorpe is a nutritionist (nutritionyoudesign.com) who suffered from fibroids for 10 years and saw 21 doctors before finally finding one who could solve her heavy bleeding without performing a hysterectomy.

> I suffered with fibroids for more than 10 years and no one was able to really help me without suggesting I have a hysterectomy or simply bleed to death, as one doctor told me. I cannot tell you how frustrated I was to hear this. I became severely anemic and my organs were starting to shut down. I was heading to death's door if something was not done. I was at the end of my rope when my aunt was able to help me find a doctor who was familiar with the right way of treating me. I had 16 fibroids, with one the size of a football.

> I had a myomectomy, which was successful, thank God. After my surgery, I realized that with better nutrition and lifestyle I could heal my own body. This is what prompted me to become a nutritionist to help other women who are battling this and other similar problems.

> Since then I have learned how to stay healthy by eating the right things to keep me fibroid-free. It has been three years since the surgery and so far so good. I would encourage women to stay positive, exercise, eat right and take a more holistic approach as there is hope out there, especially with alternative, holistic health methods.

For many younger women, the procedure holds a much deeper, more profound promise – the chance to become pregnant and have a family. When I set out to write this book, I thought I was targeting my message at women in their 30s, 40s and 50s because statistically speaking, HMB tends to most affect women in that age group. Since then, through the magic of Facebook and my website, I have heard from many women in their 20s who were faced with the same shocking news that I was – that hysterectomy was the only cure for their HMB.

Here are the stories of two of those women, Shannon from Ottawa, Ontario, and Sarah, from Rosemount, Minnesota, both 30. If you or someone you know is struggling to preserve fertility while battling fibroids, I strongly suggest you read these stories and pass them along. They will open your eyes to a whole new world of possibilities. (There are photos of Shannon and Sarah on my website, unhysterectomy.com).

Shannon

My name is Shannon, I'm 30 years old and I'm sharing my story to give other women the benefit of my experience – and to give them hope.

In 2006, I started having extremely painful and heavy periods. They got worse and worse every month, until it got to the point where I was changing my supplies every two hours and taking pain killers around the clock. I wore a super-plus tampon and an extra-thick pad, but nothing seemed to contain my flow.

I had just started seeing my future husband, Matt. One evening he invited me to meet some of his friends for the first time. I was excited, but I was also nervous because I had my period; I knew it would be a risky evening. Luckily, everything went fine - until I stood up to get my coat at the end of the evening. All I could see was a big red stain on the white upholstered chair I'd been sitting in all evening. I was mortified.

I asked my doctor what was going on. Examining me, she found a large lump in my lower abdomen. Of course, I started to worry. She sent me for an ultrasound. It was inconclusive, so she sent me to an oncologist for more tests. By this time, I was in a complete panic, thinking I had cancer. Luckily, the tests were negative for cancer, but neither doctor could say what was growing in my belly. They just sort of left me hanging, without any sort of plan to move ahead.

My aunt, who's a nurse, wasn't happy about the way I'd been treated. She started making phone calls and after much persistence, got me a referral to a gynecologist. After another ultrasound, the gynecologist diagnosed fibroids and said she could try to perform a myomectomy – she would go in through my belly and physically cut out the mass. But she said there was still a high risk of me needing a hysterectomy. Just hearing the word "hysterectomy" was enough to make me lose it. By this time Matt and I were engaged and we knew we wanted children. I walked away from the appointment feeling like I'd just found out I was infertile. I was in a daze. I remember sitting by my living room window, watching strollers go by, and just crying my eyes out.

But as luck would have it, Dr. Sony Singh had just moved to Ottawa to become the Director of Minimally Invasive Gynecology at the Shirley E. Greenberg Women's Health Centre. My first gynecologist referred me to him. From the moment we met Dr. Singh, Matt and I knew things were going to be different. Dr. Singh said he could absolutely help us without giving me a hysterectomy. I think I started crying right there in the office. We were overjoyed.

Dr. Singh told us to wait a year after my treatment before trying to have a baby, which we did. And then we got pregnant almost right away. On January 29, 2009, we were married in Jamaica; I was seven months pregnant. It was a dream come true. Two months later, our son Hudson was born. Wynston was born in April 2011.

I know there's a chance my fibroids could grow back, but I'm willing to take that chance. Now that I know there are options, I'm sure we'll be able to handle the problem without major surgery.

Whether you're 30, 40 or 50, you don't have to settle for invasive major operations. This is 2012; you have options. Even if you're done having children, or don't plan on having them, there are ways to stop your abnormal bleeding without a hysterectomy. Our two beautiful children are living proof.

Now, meet Sarah, another young woman who was told she needed a hysterectomy.

Sarah

My name is Sarah, and I am a very active and healthy 30-year-old woman who has type 1 diabetes that is very well controlled. I would like to share my personal story of my 35 uterine fibroids and the choice I made.

My journey started quite some time ago as I always complained of excessive menstrual bleeding and severe cramping at my annual exams but my gynecologist never took me seriously. During my annual pap exam in November 2011, I once again raised my concerns about my very heavy bleeding (bleeding through a super-plus tampon within a minute of insertion and wearing thick pads), severe cramping leaving me unable to stand at times, frequent urination, lower back pain and legs falling asleep frequently. It was getting to the point that I didn't want to leave the house during my cycle. I felt terrible having to cancel plans during my cycle but felt I could not tell people why due to the fear of them not believing how bad my periods really were.

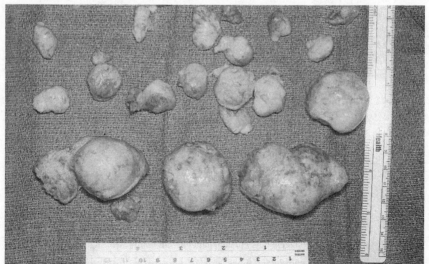

Photo courtesy of the patient.

This photo shows the fibroids removed from Sarah's uterus during her myomectomy.

During my pelvic exam, my gynecologist told me she was having a hard time reaching my cervix and that my abdomen felt enlarged. She said she wanted me to have a vaginal ultrasound and gave no explanation. I ended up going to the hospital a few days later to have the ultrasound because I was bleeding so much and feeling very weak. My gynecologist would not get back to me with my results, even after I called her office multiple times and spoke with the clinic administrator. I was very nervous and afraid and wanted to know what was going on with my body. I couldn't believe I was being brushed off by someone who was supposed to be there to care for women. I ended up getting a copy of the report from medical records, and went to an independent gynecology clinic for a second opinion.

The gynecologist I saw for my second opinion has been practicing for many years. He looked at my ultrasound report and told me things were not good. He did a pelvic exam and then explained that I had diffuse uterine fibroids, that my uterus was very distorted and that I would never be able to get pregnant or carry a child. I was alone at my appointment and this was the most devastating news of my life. I left the appointment crying and with a feeling of deep sadness and depression.

I have been married two and a half years and wanted more than anything to be pregnant. The doctor also told me an MRI could be done but he wasn't hopeful. I requested the MRI and went to him afterward for the results. He told me my condition was severe and that he had never seen anything like it in someone my age. He said surgery was not an option because it would destroy my entire uterus and that there was no specialist who could treat my condition. He said he could start me on Lupron injections (GnRH-a therapy) to try to shrink the fibroids or I could have a hysterectomy.

I didn't agree with these options but held out hope. I did my own research and found Dr. Elizabeth Stewart at the Mayo Clinic. Her recommendation was that because of the number of fibroids, the size and position of my uterus and my desire to preserve fertility, focused ultrasound was not the best option, but that she could perform an abdominal myomectomy.

On December 28, 2011, Dr. Stewart performed my myomectomy and removed 35 fibroids. She also did a D&C (dilation and curettage) to remove a polyp and removed an adhesion from the posterior portion of my uterus.

She said my surgery went very well and is hopeful for a future pregnancy. I would have liked to have had a procedure that was non- or minimally invasive and would have liked to do MR-guided focused ultrasound. Dr. Stewart said that because of my particular situation, open abdominal myomectomy was my best option. She did have to make a low horizontal bikini cut incision in order to have my uterus out and exposed to be able to see it and feel it to remove all of the fibroids. She made a vertical incision up the front part of my uterus and removed 20 fibroids, and then a vertical incision up the back part of my uterus to remove the remaining 15 fibroids. I was in the hospital for three days and am off work for six weeks. Having the open abdominal myomectomy made for a longer recovery but I was just so happy that something could be done.

I couldn't be more thankful to Dr. Stewart and her caring manner and tremendous skill in performing my operation. I am five weeks post op and I feel like I have more energy and am getting around much easier. I can't wait until the days ahead when I am fully recovered and can experience a better quality of life. It is still hard for me to believe that all those fibroids were growing inside me. I now understand why I was in so much pain. I do plan on having children once I give my body time to heal and was trying before I was diagnosed.

Dr. Stewart told me the best thing for me to help prevent the fibroids from coming back would be to carry a pregnancy. She even seemed very hopeful for me to be able to have a vaginal delivery. I feel truly blessed that Dr. Stewart and her expertise came into my life. My journey has led me to share my story with others and to let other women know not to give up and keep searching until you find a treatment choice that is right for you.

What does this all mean?

As with everything else you've read in this book, the information I've presented in this chapter about myomectomies is worth considerable thought. One drawback to the procedure is that fibroids can grow back and the risk of scarring is important to consider if future pregnancy is desired, but if you're willing to take the risk, then the surgery just might be what you're looking for.

And if you're 30 instead of 50, there may be many more alternatives to hysterectomy by the time you're that age that haven't even been invented yet! So it might be worth holding out. But again, the choice is entirely yours.

One thing I do know – and this has been mentioned repeatedly by every expert I have interviewed – is that the more women ask for these minimally invasive procedures, the more likely they are to be offered. Any economist will tell you it's a simple matter of supply and demand. It's happened with gallbladders, so why can't it happen with benign growths such as fibroids, polyps and cysts?

"Laparoscopic cholecystectomy (removal of the gallbladder), introduced in 1989 *after* laparoscopic myomectomy, is now the surgical treatment of choice rather than open cholecystectomy. The majority of American surgeons (81 percent) had adopted the procedure by 1992 and in Ontario, the number of cholecystectomies performed laparoscopically increased from 1.0 percent to 85.6 percent between 1990 and 1994."[105]

So even though laparoscopic myomectomy was developed *before* laparoscopic cholecystectomy, and even though laparoscopy has become the surgery of first resort for gallbladder removal, some 25 years later doctors are still debating the issue in relation to myomectomy.

"Canadian surgeons who perform laparoscopic myomectomy are unsure about outcomes with respect to fertility, uterine rupture risk, and myoma recurrence when laparoscopic myomectomy is compared with abdominal myomectomy," concluded the 2010 survey of Canadian gynecologists regarding myomectomy. "This makes counselling a patient difficult. Further appropriately

---

[105] Grace Liu, Lynne Zolis, Rose Kung, Mary Melchior, Sukhbir Singh and Francis Cook, "The Laparoscopic Myomectomy: A Survey of Canadian Gynecologists," *Journal of Obstetrics and Gynaecology Canada*, 147.

sized randomized controlled trials comparing laparoscopic myomectomy and abdominal myomectomy are needed. The existing evidence indicates, however, that when the procedure is performed by a properly trained surgeon, the complication rate of laparoscopic myomectomy should be low and the subsequent fertility rate, uterine rupture rate, and recurrence rate should be comparable to abdominal myomectomy."[106]

Again, the key appears to be training and motivation. As for the 70 percent of gynecologists who said they were unsure about who performed the procedure in Canada, or to whom to refer their patients, I would be more than happy to volunteer to research such a list and put a copy in the mail to each and every ob-gyn in Canada.

---

[106] Grace Liu, Lynne Zolis, Rose Kung, Mary Melchior, Sukhbir Singh and Francis Cook, "The Laparoscopic Myomectomy: A Survey of Canadian Gynecologists," *Journal of Obstetrics and Gynaecology Canada*, 147.

Chapter 16
Robotics

Through the magic of Facebook, I have met many new friends while writing this book. One of them is a delightful woman from Knoxville, Tennessee, named Teresa. She sent me a message out of the blue one day because I have the same name as an old friend she'd lost touch with. We got to talking and I told her I was writing a book about minimally invasive alternatives to hysterectomy. In true Southern style, this warm and friendly woman I had never met suddenly opened up to me.

"How ironic that you are researching hysterectomies for your book," she told me. "I just had one about six weeks ago. This decision was not by choice. I had uterine prolapse and it was pushing my other female parts down and out through the vagina. It was suggested by my ob-gyn that I have a complete hysterectomy as I am 53 years old, was already post-menopausal and had been for many years.

"I had five tiny incisions across my stomach parallel with my navel. They called it robotic surgery. They also had to suspend my bladder because after eight years, the muscles were too relaxed to support it. They did that vaginally. The recovery was pretty quick. Had surgery on Tuesday, came home on Wednesday, rested up Friday and Saturday and on Sunday I baked a ham, cooked pinto beans, corn bread and potatoes. Each week I got better."

Although robotics are becoming more popular in the US for everything from endometriosis surgery to hysterectomy to prostate cancer treatment, Canadian hospitals are naturally slower to adopt the technology, for obvious reasons. At $2.5 million, the robots are expensive and require aggressive fundraising by hospitals. Still, Canada must be interested in embracing robotics or the federal, provincial and territorial governments would not have funded a 298-page study on the subject.[107] As of early 2012, 11 Canadian hospitals[108] were using a robot to perform a variety of procedures, including prostatectomy, hysterectomy, nephrectomy (kidney removal) and cardiac surgery. Surgeons at St. Joseph's Health Centre in London, Ontario, performed Canada's first robotic-assisted radical hysterectomy in 2008.[109]

Are six hands better than two?

Da Vinci robots are the most widely marketed and studied surgical robots in the world and the only ones approved for use in Canada.[110] With the Da Vinci, despite what you may envision, the surgeon is the master while the robot is the servant. The surgeon still controls the surgery, but from a computer station a few feet away from the patient. His or her hands never touch the patient, except to insert the initial laparoscopes.

"The robotic platform arises from the laparoscopic platform, which is a minimally invasive surgical approach so we don't really open up the abdomen, we make small incisions," says Dr. Neena Agarwala, a gynecologist from State College, Pennsylvania, who trains gynecologists from around the world in the Da Vinci procedure. I met her at the 40th Annual Global Congress on Minimally Invasive Gynecology in Hollywood, Florida, in November 2011. The congress was organized by the leading professional society for advanced laparoscopy in the world, the

---

[107] Canadian Agency for Drugs and Technologies in Health, "Robot-Assisted Surgery Compared with Open Surgery and Laparoscopic Surgery: Clinical Effectiveness and Economic Analyses," CADTH Technology Report no. 137 (Sept. 2011).

[108] Canadian Agency for Drugs and Technologies in Health. "Robot-Assisted Surgery Compared with Open Surgery and Laparoscopic Surgery: Clinical Effectiveness and Economic Analyses," 2.

[109] St. Joseph's Health Centre, "Robotic Assisted Radical Hysterectomy a Canadian First – The Breakthrough Is a Boon to Women with Cervical Cancer," 2008. News release.

[110] Canadian Agency for Drugs and Technologies in Health. "Robot-Assisted Surgery Compared with Open Surgery and Laparoscopic Surgery: Clinical Effectiveness and Economic Analyses," 14.

American Association of Gynecological Laparoscopists (AAGL). The Canadian Society of Minimally Invasive Gynecology is one of a number of new professional medical societies that are springing up around the world in response to the need for training and advocacy.

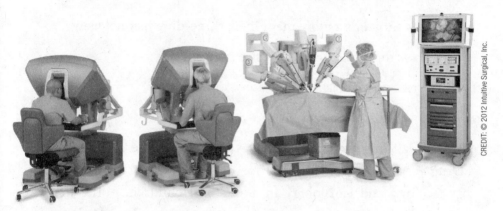

The full Da Vinci surgical system.

"The first instrument we insert via a small incision is a camera or a laparoscope, which then becomes our eyes and this view is then projected on a screen, Dr. Agarwala explained. "We operate by looking at the screen as if we were looking straight into the abdomen and then we use our hands to 'perform' the task that we are intending to perform."

With the Da Vinci, between four and six laparoscopes are inserted into the area of the body requiring the surgery; in the case of hysterectomy, it's the upper and lower abdomen. The surgeon sits at the computer console watching a monitor that projects a live 3-D picture coming from the scopes inside the patient. Using manoeuvrable handles, the surgeon tells the robot what to do.

The Da Vinci is said to be better than traditional surgery because it:

- Reduces physician fatigue

- Requires a smaller surgical team in the operating room

- Requires smaller incisions

- Gives surgeons a more magnified, three-dimensional view

- Allows for more minute, precise movements

- Carries a lower risk of infection

- Allows faster recovery

The Da Vinci surgical system was approved by the US Food and Drug Administration in 2000 for urology, general laparoscopy, gynecology and cardiology in adults and children.[111] The first-generation Da Vinci Surgical System (the Da Vinci Standard) was approved by Health Canada in March 2001. Since then, second- and third-generation Da Vinci robots have been approved.

I had the opportunity to watch Dr. Agarwala training surgeons during the AAGL global congress and it was fascinating. Imagine a large hotel ballroom filled with surgeons in scrubs, sitting in front of giant computer consoles, with rows of cadavers on operating tables beside them. I made a video of the training session, which you can see on my website.

"The robotic platform has enhanced the laparoscopic platform in two ways – one, it projects a three-dimensional view, which gives the surgeon a sense of immersion into that part of the patient we are working on; and secondly, the instruments have better ergonomics and movement at the wrist, which allows for a

---

[111] Canadian Agency for Drugs and Technologies in Health. "Robot-Assisted Surgery Compared with Open Surgery and Laparoscopic Surgery: Clinical Effectiveness and Economic Analyses," 2.

360° rotation of the tips of the instrument rather than a straight rigid approach to the tissue."

It was obvious from watching Dr. Agarwala, who is part of a network of Canadian and US gynecologists who work closely together through their AAGL connection, that she is passionate about minimally invasive gynecology.

> I am particularly passionate about laparoscopic and robotic surgery because I really think, if I may say, women are an essential part of our society and our households. I really believe that taking care of women in a minimally invasive fashion really has a very positive outcome on our society. It affects our workforce and our family force. If a mother is down for six weeks, it really puts a strain on her family and her work environment so if I can take care of a woman's ailment or disease, and yet return her to her functioning capacity within two weeks, it's very hard to measure that societal cost, but I think it can make a huge impact on how our society functions.
>
> So I am particularly excited about minimally invasive surgery because I deal with women and I feel women deserve the best. By providing this minimally invasive surgical platform it really does help educate and provide services to women who would otherwise forgo care for themselves in favour of work and family. Women often don't take care of themselves because they think they don't have the time to be down for six weeks, so I really think I make a huge difference in their lives and that gives me extreme pleasure and satisfaction.

Is robotic surgery the way of the future?

We pretty much know that robotics are here to stay, but are they really that much better than traditional surgery done by human hands? Using the silk purse/sow's ear analogy, some doctors I have spoken with believe that all the bells and whistles in the world cannot make a great surgeon out of an average one. Is it a turf war between man and machine, ego and the cold hard truth? Perhaps it's all of that. One thing is for sure: initial studies are pointing to the need for more studies. A 2012 report in the *Journal of Clinical Oncology*[112] found similar complication rates among women who had laparoscopic or robotic hysterectomies for endometrial cancer.

"Despite claims of decreased complications with robotic hysterectomy, we found similar morbidity but increased cost compared with laparoscopic hysterectomy," researchers concluded. "Comparative long-term efficacy data are needed to justify its widespread use."

Dr. Parker agrees. In fact, he fears robotics may be worse for women, not better.

Robotic surgery is kind of the new thing and probably not necessary at this point. What I think is going to happen is that since it's easier for the doctor to do a robotic hysterectomy they might forego offering women simpler other alternatives like the Mirena IUD, endometrial ablation, laparoscopic myomectomy or a host of other things. I'm afraid of that. Robotics make the doctor seem sexy and on the cutting edge, but it's really not in the patient's best interest.

If you're not a good surgeon and you don't know the anatomy and you have bad technique the robot's not helping. And they're starting to see that. They're seeing poor patient selection. They're seeing complications. We have to have better criteria for selecting patients more appropriately and screening out the surgeons who don't have the expertise to be doing this kind of surgery. The bottom line is if you're offered a robotic hysterectomy, it's still a hysterectomy. It's no different. It's just a different instrument. I think every woman should be asking "What are my alternatives? How many cases have you done like mine clinically? What have the results been? What kind of complications have you had?"

---

[112] Jason D. Wright, William M. Burke, Elizabeth T. Wilde, Sharyn N. Lewin, Abigail S. Charles, Jin Hee Kim, Noah Goldman et al., "Comparative Effectiveness of Robotic Versus Laparoscopic Hysterectomy for Endometrial Cancer," *Journal of Clinical Oncology* (Feb. 2012) e-pub ahead of print.

Women need to be able to evaluate the person who's going to be operating on them. That's a big deal. One of my patients said to me the definition of minor surgery is surgery happening to somebody else. I totally agree with that. You know, the robot sounds better but there are some dangers that we know about and there are some dangers that we don't even know about yet. As I said before, if you can do minimally invasive procedures that are less deforming to a woman's body, why not do that first?

Whatever the future holds, there is philosophical food for thought to be had by glancing back to the namesake of all of this, Leonardo da Vinci, the 15th century Renaissance philosopher, inventor, architect, engineer, mathematician and artist who painted the *Mona Lisa* and *The Last Supper*. "Where the spirit does not work with the hand, there is no art," he said. Does that mean that a robot with no spirit cannot perform great surgery? There are heady questions ahead for patients, and for surgeons who for centuries have prided themselves on their surgical technique. Can robots ever really replace surgeons? Maybe; maybe not, depending on whether you believe medicine is an art or a science.

"Medicine is an art as well as a science," says Dr. Toub of Gynesonics. "And sometimes it's a little more art than science."

Chapter 17
How to Access These Procedures No Matter Where You Live

Whether you live in rural or urban Canada, accessing minimally invasive gynecology is a challenge. Yes, your chance of accessing this type of surgery is greater if you live near a major centre, preferably one with a teaching hospital, but in reality, even major Canadian cities have fewer gynecologists who specialize in this important sub-speciality than they should. My heart goes out to women in rural areas, who are doubly challenged.

Whenever I think of rural women I think of Bernice MacDonald. I met Bernice when I was living on Prince Edward Island in the early 1990s. I was doing a series of stories for CBC Television on Island traditions and somehow caught wind of this stubborn, white-haired, self-proclaimed "tomboy" who insisted on riding her bicycle into town rather than drive. I can hear her deep, crackling voice as if it were yesterday. When I went to visit Bernice at her little white house in Chepstow, near Souris, overlooking Northumberland Strait, she gave me a tour of her garden and gave me some of the wild blueberries she loved to eat. She stooped down to pick some and slipped them into the palm of my hand.

"Look at the bee-ute-ee-ful hands you young girls have nowadays," she croaked, extending her dry, cracked hands while checking mine for calluses. You may be wondering what this has to do with this book, but it has everything to do with this book. Hysterectomy rates for rural women in Canada are 46 percent higher than for women in urban areas. Part of that is obviously due to a shortage of doctors, but also when you live in small towns like Chepstow, PEI, away from a major centre, life is different, quieter, with fewer things to choose from and longer distances to travel for things like groceries and doctor's appointments. I remember travelling four and a half hours to Halifax from Charlottetown for allergy testing because there were no allergists on the Island. It never occurred to me that it was any big deal.

Healthcare 101

In 1911, the Douglas family was preparing to move from Scotland to Canada when their young son Tommy fell and injured his right knee. Infection set in and the boy underwent a number of surgeries in Scotland to prevent the infection from spreading. After the family settled in Winnipeg, Tommy's bone infection flared up again and the boy was sent to hospital. Doctors told his parents his leg would have to be amputated. The family was poor and worried about how they would pay for such an operation. A local orthopedic surgeon took an interest in the case and offered to treat the boy for free if his students could watch. After several surgeries, the boy's leg was saved, but the experience stayed with him. As you are no doubt aware, Tommy Douglas went on to create the first provincial healthcare plan in Canadian history.[113]

"I felt that no boy should have to depend either for his leg or his life upon the ability of his parents to raise enough money to bring a first class surgeon to his bedside,"[114] Douglas said. As premier of Saskatchewan, he introduced provincial hospital insurance in 1947, which led to the introduction of Medicare in Saskatchewan in 1962 by his successor, Woodrow Lloyd. "I'm sure that the standard of public morality we've helped build will force government in Canada to approve complete health insurance," Douglas said in a 1958 interview. By 1961, every province and territory had public insurance plans that provided universal access to hospital services.

[113] Canadian Museum of Civilization, "Making Medicare: The History of Health Care in Canada , 1914-2007," 2012, http://www.civilization.ca/cmc/exhibitions/hist/medicare/medic-3g03e.shtml.
[114] Lewis H. Thomas, ed. *The Making of a Socialist: The Recollections of T. C. Douglas* (Edmonton: University of Alberta Press, 1982), 7.

In 1966, the federal government had passed the *Medical Care Act* to begin sharing the cost of insuring physician services with the provinces and territories. By 1972, all provincial and territorial plans had been extended to include physician services.[115] After a review of healthcare in 1979, and a lengthy national debate, the *Canada Health Act* came into being in 1984.

What this means for Canadian patients

Although we have a national law governing the provision of healthcare services in Canada, we actually have no national health plan. The Canadian health insurance system is delivered through 13 provincial and territorial health insurance plans, the mandate of which "ensure[s] that all eligible residents of Canada have reasonable access to medically necessary hospital and physician services."[116]

The *Canada Health Act* has five criteria, which all provincial and territorial health plans must satisfy to receive the health transfer payments from the federal government that pays for our care as patients:

1. Public administration

2. Portability

3. Accessibility

4. Universality

5. Comprehensiveness

To provide equal access to healthcare for all Canadians, section 12a of the *Canada Health Act* states that provincial health insurance plans must "Provide for insured health services on

---

[115] Health Canada, "Annual Report 2009/2010: Introduction," 2010, www.hc-sc.gc.ca (accessed 2012).
[116] Justice Canada, *Canada Health Act*, www.laws-lois.justice.gc.ca/eng/acts/C-6.

uniform terms and conditions and on a basis that does not impede or preclude, either directly or indirectly whether by charges made to insured persons or otherwise, reasonable access to those services by insured persons."

So *in theory*, whether you live in Chepstow, PEI, or Wynyard, Saskatchewan, you have the right to the same level of care as every other Canadian. So does that mean that if Wynyard doesn't have a gynecologist who can perform a myomectomy instead of a hysterectomy you can sue the federal government for violating the terms of the act? I'm not a lawyer, but from what I understand, you have the right to ask for *prior permission* from your provincial health ministry to travel to another province to have the procedure done. Whether or not your expenses would be paid by your home province is a matter of negotiation between you and your health insurance plan.

Here is what the *Canada Health Act* states regarding accessibility and portability. I have highlighted the relevant passages in bold:

4. Portability (section 11)

Residents moving from one province or territory to another must continue to be covered for insured health services by the "home" jurisdiction during any waiting period imposed by the new province or territory of residence. The waiting period for eligibility to a provincial or territorial health care insurance plan must not exceed three months. After the waiting period, the new province or territory of residence assumes responsibility for health care coverage. However, it is the responsibility of residents to inform their province or territory's health care insurance plan that they are leaving and to register with the health care insurance plan of their new province or territory.

Residents who are temporarily absent from their home province or territory or from Canada, must continue to be covered for insured health services during their absence. This allows individuals to travel or be absent from their home province or territory, within a prescribed duration, while retaining their health insurance coverage.

The portability criterion does not entitle a person to seek services in another province, territory or country, but is intended to permit a person to receive necessary services in relation to an urgent or emergent need when absent on a temporary basis, such as on business or vacation.

If insured persons are temporarily absent in another province or territory, the portability criterion requires that insured services be paid at the host province's rate. If insured persons are temporarily out of the country, insured services are to be paid at the home province's rate.

Prior approval by the health care insurance plan in a person's home province or territory may also be required before coverage is extended for elective (non-emergency) services to a resident while temporarily absent from his/her province or territory.

5. Accessibility (section 12)

The intent of the accessibility criterion is to ensure that insured persons in a province or territory have **reasonable access** to insured hospital, medical and surgical-dental services **on uniform terms and conditions**, unprecluded or unimpeded, either directly or indirectly, by charges (user charges or extra-billing) or other means (e.g., discrimination on the basis of age, health status or financial circumstances).

In addition, the health care insurance plans of the province or territory must provide:

- Reasonable compensation to physicians and dentists for all the insured health services they provide; and payment to hospitals to cover the cost of insured health services.

Reasonable access in terms of physical availability of medically necessary services has been interpreted under the Canada Health Act using the "where and as available" rule. Thus, residents of a province or territory are entitled to have access on uniform terms and conditions to insured health services at the setting "where" the services are provided and "as" the services are available in that setting.[117]

---

[117] Health Canada. *Canada Health Act Annual Report 2010-1011*.
www.hc-sc.gc.ca/hcs-sss/pubs/cha-lcs/2011-cha-lcs-ar-ra/index-eng.php#chap1.

Does that mean, for instance, that if you live in Sarnia or Thunder Bay and you want to travel to Ottawa for a surgery that is not readily available in your area that the Ontario Health Insurance Plan would conceivably pay for that? It very well might, according to my research. Provincial health plans are set up to help people so if you live in a remote or rural area where medical services are limited, you could ask your doctor to refer you to a specialist outside of your hometown in order to gain the necessary prior approval from your provincial health plan.

All provincial healthcare plans, except Quebec's, have reciprocal billing agreements for hospital physicians. So if you have a medical emergency in another province, your provincial health card is all you need to show to have your treatment covered. Non-emergency medical treatments, for things such as laparoscopic hysterectomy, laparoscopic myomectomy and hysteroscopic endometrial ablations, are a whole other kettle of fish.

You need to know before you undertake treatment whether or not your provincial healthcare plan is willing to cover your procedure. When you are seeking services outside your province, whether it's in another part of Canada or outside of Canada, prior approval is a *must*. Because if you don't get prior approval then essentially you're taking things into your own hands and you'd be responsible for the costs that you incurred.

Your plan of attack

Based on everything you've learned in this book, if there's a procedure you think might help but that's not offered in your area, I suggest you follow these five steps:

1. **Identify the procedure you want.** Discuss your options with your family doctor or gynecologist and try to have the procedure done close to home. If the procedure is not available

within a reasonable distance, or the waiting list is ridiculously long, move on to the next step.

2. **Contact your provincial healthcare system.** Ask if the plan will cover your costs if you travel either somewhere within your home province or to another province. If the answer is yes, or even maybe, ask what you need to do to gain *prior approval* for the procedure and do it. If the answer is no, contact your member of provincial parliament and ask what you should do next. Go online and search for precedents where other patients in your area have received prior approval for certain surgeries. Download anything you can find that may establish a precedent that you can benefit from.

3. **Establish a paper trail.** Keep records of who you speak with and what they said and save all your emails. Also, get as much diagnostic proof as you can from your family doctor or your gynecologist to demonstrate the severity of your condition: ultrasounds, blood work, MRIs, etc. Ask for copies of test results and reports and keep them in a safe place. Use the tools previously discussed to push for the tests and documentation you need. Just like a good lawyer, you're *building a case* for yourself as to why your condition requires faster, better care than you can get at home.

4. **Try to work with your doctors, not against them.** Many doctors are as frustrated as we are, so you may be surprised at how helpful they may be. Unless their ego gets in the way, most doctors are willing to do whatever they can to help their patients get well.

5. **Go to your local media.** The media love a good story and if you feel you're being discriminated against in any way by being denied equal access to equal care, then say it in an interview. Ask

the reporter to call your member of provincial parliament and request a statement on why you were denied access. Remember, Canada is paying millions of dollars to send patients to the US every year for care that is not available here. The only way we are ever going to have coverage for out-of-province or out-of-country treatment for menstrual disorders is by asking.

Women from Quebec should be especially diligent in contacting their provincial health ministry as the rules for inter-provincial care are different in Quebec than in the rest of Canada.

Cross-border care

Need surgery, will travel. To illustrate just how desperate some Canadian women are for relief from their painful, heavy menstrual bleeding, I will introduce you to Lisa, a 46-year-old construction worker from Edmonton. After three years of trying to have her heavy periods and swollen belly properly diagnosed, Lisa bit the bullet and spent $25,000 of her own money to fly to California for a myomectomy. The majority of the $25,000 went towards hospital fees.

> *The situation for rural women is very different than for women who live near a major centre. Think about it. It takes six months to get an appointment with a gynecologist, they live hundreds of miles away, they've got four kids and they're bleeding.. You've got one gynecologist servicing people who live very far from the major centre. In order to do a lot of this conservative therapy, it's very time consuming. So a lot of patients don't want it. Their mother had a hysterectomy, their grandmother had a hysterectomy and they were improved right away in terms of the bleeding problem. They want something fast and they want it definitive. They don't want to keep having to go back and forth or keep taking time off work. They come in and they want it fixed. So they just say, "You know what? Just fix it." On the other hand, if you live in Toronto, it's not so bad just to take the subway to the gynecologist."*
>
> – Dr. Wendy Wolfman, Mount Sinai Hospital, Toronto

In 2007 I realized my periods were really heavy but I had no idea what was causing it. I would wake up in the night and there was this blood all over. By the end I was using towels just to keep up with the flow. It was really hard to function. I couldn't go to work and bleed all over the construction site when all I had was a Porta-Potty. I don't know if it was stress or the work, but within a year I looked like I was four months pregnant and I had no idea why.

I told my doctor, but he just waved at me and said it was nothing and that I was just having heavy periods. He just dismissed it. It wasn't until Christmas 2009 when his receptionist happened to ask me how my fibroid was doing because it was so big, like four inches around. The doctor didn't even bother to tell me that I had a fibroid. I had never used the computer before to research health conditions but I started looking around and I came across Dr. Parker's site. I saw a video of this surgery and just said, "Wow." So I went back to my doctor and told him about it. He said he would refer me to someone in Edmonton who could help me without taking out my uterus but because it was going to take me five months to get in, I called Dr. Parker's office to see when they could get me in. They asked me to get an MRI and then they would know. When I asked my doctor about this he just sort of said, "Yeah, that's the way it is in Canada, or that's the way it's going. You're going to have to go to the States to get stuff done."

Anyway, I got the MRI and sent them the disc and Dr. Parker emailed me and said he could remove my fibroid laparoscopically without a hysterectomy. Luckily, they had a cancellation and I got in 10 days later. I had the surgery, stayed in a hotel overnight and flew back to Edmonton within a couple of days.

I had the money in the bank but that's not the point. I pay my taxes here in Canada but I had to go to the States to have surgery. I don't want to be paying double for stuff. That's the whole problem. But if I'd stayed in Canada, they might have given me a hysterectomy, which I didn't want. If I had a brain tumour, would they take out my brain? So why take out my uterus just because it has a fibroid in it? It's barbaric. It's so stupid what they're doing here. It makes no sense to me. It's violence against women. And they don't give a shit about women in society. If men had this problem, they wouldn't be doing that.

Having said that, the young, new generation give their nurses a high five when they don't do surgery. Like they're all about avoiding hysterectomy wherever possible.

Although Lisa managed to solve her heavy periods by travelling to the United States, she still doesn't feel like her old self. Her bleeding's stopped but now she's battling peri-menopause symptoms such as memory loss, interrupted sleep and fatigue that are bringing her down. At least by having a myomectomy, she's able to enter menopause naturally, but as those of us of a certain vintage know, menopause presents a whole new set of challenges.

Deciding to cross the border for medical care is a very big decision. Lisa was lucky that she didn't develop any complications. Her surgery came in at the expected $25,000 she budgeted for. But what if things don't go as planned? I've been told of women who ended up spending $100,000 because they developed complications after surgery and required more care.

"I hope those women are few and far between because surgery is expensive," says Dr. Leyland. "Our Canadian healthcare system ought to be able to offer a standard of care and appropriate interventions for all patients. Through the *Canada Health Act*, women should not have to pay out of their own pocket to find this type of treatment. Instead, we should be developing a system where we can provide the best, least invasive and least expensive types of care for women in Canada. I think it's very unfortunate that people have to actually seek care elsewhere when there are physicians in most parts of Canada who are providing this kind of intervention right now. Even the money that provincial healthcare plans do approve to send patients to the US for surgery could be kept here and used to create centres of excellence across the country to allow for a greater number of women to access a greater number of outpatient services. Women should not have to pay for it out of their own pocket."

Before making any decisions on whether to travel outside Canada for surgery, I strongly suggest you read the report *Evolving Medical Tourism in Canada. Exploring a New Frontier.*[118] It's an eye-opening report on the growing trend towards medical tourism, which at the time the report was published was expected to grow to a US$40 billion industry worldwide by 2010.

---

[118] Lisa Purdy and Mark Fam, "*Evolving Medical Tourism in Canada. Exploring a New Frontier,*" The Deloitte Center for Health Solutions, www.deloitte.com/centerforhealthsolutions.com (accessed Jan. 2012).

Chapter 18
Empowering Our Daughters

Most eye-opening moment for the mother of two teenage girls: the day my daughter came home from grade 10 complaining how "gross" it was that some girls her age were not wearing underwear beneath their school kilts. Second most eye-opening moment: the day my other daughter told me she learned about the dangers of anal sex on the last day of school before summer holiday. She was 11. Although I knew it intuitively, I now had proof of how much times have changed since my time at Dublin Public Elementary School. We're not in Kansas anymore and it's up to us, as parents, to help our children make sense of it all.

I really believe that children learn what they live, so if we, as parents, can empower our children to develop their own emotional, mental, physical and moral compass, then we can pat ourselves on the back for a job well done. We must help our daughters now to become the patients of tomorrow. Our mothers did the best they could with what they had. It was not in their nature to stand up to authority, but it is in ours. And it should be in our daughters, too.

"Hysterectomy is a glaring example [of the need to empower our daughters]," says Dr. Ashton. "I look at it as laying the foundation for how these girls are going to care for themselves and their families their entire life."

Hopefully by the time our daughters are past their childbearing years, or perhaps even before, science will have made the breakthroughs so many of us are craving now, at least where the treatment for HMB is concerned. I hope that by the time I am a grandmother, there will be no need for hysterectomies, or even less-invasive alternatives. I hope that touchless, scarless surgery becomes the standard of care for every woman. I hope by the time my children are grandmothers, HMB will be a treatable condition that does not require any kind of surgical intervention.

Seize the moment

As a mother, I truly believe that every moment is a teaching moment; what we do, think, feel or say has the power to influence our children in a most profound way. If we can be truly present with our daughters, truly engaged in what's going on in their lives by listening to the music they listen to, or watching the shows they watch (go *Gossip Girl*), reading the books they read and truly *listening* to them, we will pass on the most powerful lesson of all to them as human beings, not just as women: that they are important, they are valued and their thoughts and opinions are worth listening to. So that if, or when, they encounter a difficult situation, perhaps with a doctor, a boss, a partner or a friend, they can draw on those moments and assert themselves with power and grace.

Remember, talking about menstruation with your daughters is not quite the same as discussing sex. Talking with our daughters about their reproductive organs does not mean they're going to run out and start using them.

"One unfortunate thing is that in this country [the US] today, people equate gynecologists with sex doctors so even though you have an 11-year old who's getting a period every month, or a 14-year old who's sexually active, people don't think that those teenagers, those children, should see a gynecologist and that, in my opinion, is not the appropriate approach," says Dr. Ashton. "It has nothing to do with sex. It has to do with educating a girl about what to expect when she gets her period, what to expect as her breasts change and how to care for her body as it changes. One of the things I'll tell a 12-year old is when you get your period, if it hurts, don't say 'I have a stomach ache' because if you say that to any woman (your mom), she's going to think you're going to vomit or you have a stomach virus, but if you say you have cramps, every woman knows that what means. So that's just a very concrete example of how much empowering, enlightening information can be conveyed to a young teenager by a gynecologist and why, in my opinion, if you don't take a young girl or teenager to a gynecologist, you're missing out on an opportunity to educate her and really empower her about her health. When you have an 11-year old who's bleeding every month that can be an overwhelming physical and emotional experience. So I think that the more people you have helping her, the better."

In Canada, I doubt many family doctors would grant a referral for a teenage girl to see a gynecologist unless there was something wrong, but I think what Dr. Ashton is saying makes sense. Young girls and women need to know about what's happening to their bodies. Whether the information comes from a family doctor, a gynecologist, a pediatrician, a nurse practitioner or a text message that you send to your daughter at school, the key is to *communicate*. I remember vividly when my daughters were in grade 8 and I was asked to give my consent for them to be immunized against human papillomavirus (HPV), the virus that can cause cervical cancer. It was one of those moments when I realized just how important mother-daughter communication really is.

I have heard from so many women who say their problems started from the day they got their first period. They wish they knew then what they know now. Let's teach our daughters what we know now. We know that endometriosis is now being diagnosed in girls as young as 12, because of breakthrough technology and diagnostics. We also know that adolescent girls require a much different kind of care than adult women because of the many changes that are occurring within their bodies and the unprecedented societal pressures they face nowadays. Many things can cause abnormal uterine bleeding in adolescents so it pays to be aware and stay connected with your daughters.

Vaginal bleeding is considered abnormal in adolescents if:

- It occurs outside of the normal menstrual cycle (i.e., between periods)

- It is heavy or painful enough to disrupt their quality of life

- It stops (i.e., pregnancy)

Bleeding in a girl who has not begun to menstruate could be a sign of something more serious, or sexual abuse.

There are many causes of abnormal vaginal bleeding in adolescents, including:

- Emotional stress

- Hormonal imbalances caused by conditions such as hypothyroidism (an underactive thyroid) or diabetes

- Benign conditions such as fibroids, polyps, cysts or endometriosis

- Infection of pelvic organs, sometimes caused by sexually transmitted diseases

- Childbirth or abortion

If your daughter complains of terrible cramps and heavy bleeding, or seems to be suffering in silence, *please* have her checked. Ask your family doctor for a referral to a gynecologist who specializes in adolescent gynecology. Although they can be hard to find, they are out there. In Canada, adolescent gynecology is a growing sub-speciality within the field of gynecology, which bodes well for the treatment of abnormal vaginal bleeding in young women. Dr. Ashton says it's taken a long time for adolescent gynecology to gain acceptance.

In the past, most people thought there wasn't a lot difference between what befalls women and adolescent girls, so there was no need for a specialized fellowship or training program in the field of adolescent gynecology. But it is much harder for teenage girls now than ever before.

I really kind of fell in love with that age group when I was doing my residency training in New York City. I took care of a 13-year-old girl who we had operated on and she actually wound up needing to have one of her ovaries removed. She had a large cyst that was more than 10 centimetres and it had twisted the blood supply to the ovary. It had been misdiagnosed by other doctors so by the time she presented to our hospital, the ovary was completely dead and needed to be removed. And when I saw the way the surgical team, of which I was a part, took care of her I really thought it was very wrong. They treated her the same way they would have treated a 23-year-old, a 33-year-old, a 43-year-old and without any regard for her developmental age group. I was already a mother at that point so that might have had something to do with it, but I just thought that it was medically and philosophically kind of suboptimal to do that. So I joined a society called NASPAG, which stands for the North American Society for Pediatric and Adolescent Gynecology, and I started attending their yearly meetings, which are very small. There are only about 300 or 400 people who attend these meetings and a lot of them come from Canada, actually. I would say maybe 10 to 15 percent of the attendees of this society and these meetings are Canadian. About 75 percent of them are gynecologists while the rest are pediatricians or nurse practitioners.

I really started to self-educate in this field and this age group and as with many things, the more I learned, the more patients I saw and word got out among pediatricians and parents and teenagers and I'm so proud and happy to say that today, the under 21-year-old age group represents exactly 50 percent of my practice. It's a real privilege to be a partner with a woman or girl through the majority of her lifetime and that's exactly what I wanted to do.

In fact, Dr. Ashton's passion for caring for adolescent girls is what prompted her to write her first book, *The Body Scoop for Girls*. The book covers everything from breast development and nipple bumps, to birth control, eating disorders and hair removal "down there."

"The book is really meant to be a handbook, a head-to-toe guide for both teenagers and their parents in that 10- to 21-year old age group because I feel like that's a unique decade and it really does deserve a unique approach. It shouldn't be a one-size-fits-all in terms of telling girls, 'You have a uterus and ovaries, so I'm going to treat you like I treat a 30-year old.'"

Resources

There are a few places you can go for more information that may prove very helpful in the chats with your daughter. The Society of Obstetricians and Gynecologists of Canada has developed two very good websites – sexualityandu.ca and endometriosisinfo.ca – and the American Congress of Obstetricians and Gynecologists has developed some very good tools; do an Internet search for "adolescent sexuality and sex education." Dr. Ashton's book Body Scoop for Girls is another fabulous resource. It should be required reading for every mom and every daughter.

The saying goes that youth is wasted on the young. Let's try to prevent our daughters from wasting their youth writhing in pain or staying home during their periods. Let's teach them everything we can about what's normal and not normal about the way they bleed every month so that when they're our age, they won't have to read books like this. They'll just know what to do. These are the most wondrous years of their lives and it's our duty as mothers to see that it stays that way.

Epilogue

The subject of hysterectomy has the power to spark conversations among women in a way that few other medical subjects can, aside from childbirth, abortion and maybe breast augmentation. Such discussions break down walls between women of all incomes, all ethnic backgrounds, all political stripes and social strata who might otherwise have little to say to each other. Almost every woman I meet has a story to tell about hysterectomy, whether it's about herself or someone she knows. Not every woman gets cancer, but by God we all get periods.

I ran into a federal cabinet minister in the building where I rented an office to write this book. We shared the elevator ride from the ground floor to the 11th. In the time it took to ride that elevator, I learned more about her life than she probably realized. We shared the usual pleasantries until I told her about the book. "My sister had a hysterectomy at 24. Heavy bleeding," she said softly. "Sad, isn't it?"

It is sad and that is precisely why I wrote this book. The time for sadness is past. The time for action is now. Our healthcare system is on the verge of collapse and the money we are wasting in hospital operating rooms has simply got to be saved. Canadian women deserve the right treatment for their conditions at the right time in the right place and our gynecologists deserve to be more fairly and equitably compensated for the services they provide.

The solution is about value, not volume. It's about leveraging technology and embracing innovation. It's about reigning in spending and ramping up common sense.

The conclusion of the Mowat Centre's report "Fiscal Sustainability and the Transformation of Canada's Health Care System. A Shifting Gears Report"[119] sums it up beautifully:

> Current rates of growth in government spending on healthcare are not sustainable. This report has outlined a framework that suggests there is hope that costs can be brought down. Canadian government investments over the past decade have established a platform on which we can harvest the productivity gains from these investments. The result is a transformation in our healthcare system, facilitated by technology.
>
> Policy makers are increasingly seeing healthcare as the high-tech industry that it is. Regulations, pricing, and administrative models will need to catch up to reflect this. This new lens through which governments are seeing healthcare represents a significant change from traditional approaches. It creates huge opportunities to improve access and quality for patients, without increasing costs.
>
> Key changes occurring include the use of disruptive technologies, huge productivity and efficiency gains in some practice areas, improved quality in some procedures without increased cost, and new forms of compensation. Policy makers are finding ways to encourage these evolutions.
>
> General hospitals may be broken up to allow innovation to occur. Virtualization of healthcare will expand. How practitioners are compensated should evolve. The pricing and regulatory environment will be challenged to keep up with real time changes that take place far more quickly than traditional administrative processes can move.
>
> This policy discussion has nothing to do with current debates over alternative ways of channelling more money into the healthcare system through higher taxes, user fees, or more for-profit care. Those debates distract us away from what is really going on: a technological revolution in healthcare that holds open the promise of reigning in the growth in healthcare spending in a manner consistent with the

---

[119] W. Falk, M. Mendelsohn and J. Hjartson, *Fiscal Sustainability and the Transformation of Canada's Health Care System. A Shifting Gears Report* (Toronto: Mowat Centre/of Public Policy and Governance, University of Toronto, 2011), 50.

Canada Health Act – if policy makers, practitioners, and patients manage this clutch moment properly.

My vision for seizing that "clutch moment":

- Increase access for Canadian women to the least-invasive, most cost-effective gynecological procedures no matter where they live, how much they earn or how old they are

- Make Canadians more aware of the mental, physical, emotional and financial toll that HMB takes on women, their families and our society

- Inspire a national dialogue on the appropriateness of care, or lack thereof, given to Canadian women for the treatment of HMB

- Lobby provincial governments to see the cost savings that are possible by taking the treatment of painful, heavy menstrual bleeding out of operating rooms and into the community through the establishment of publically funded, community-based outpatient clinics across Canada, similar to those that have been set up for bariatric surgery

- Lobby provincial healthcare insurance plans to offer financial incentives to gynecologists for performing minimally invasive surgery

- Lobby the federal government to introduce legislation making pre-hysterectomy counselling mandatory in Canada

- Raise funds for the creation of the first national Chair in Minimally Invasive Gynecology; such a chair would be solely dedicated to researching abnormal uterine, and heavy menstrual, bleeding, advancing the development of state-of-the-art treatments, raising public awareness and training the physicians of tomorrow

- And finally, to put a green daisy on the lapel of every man, woman and child in this country to raise awareness and funds to help these initiatives become a reality. My dream is to make green daisies the new pink ribbons, but there's much work to do.

Will you join me?

Visit unhysterectomy.com.

Resources

PROVINCIAL HEALTH DEPARTMENTS

Alberta Health and Wellness
Box 1360, Station Main
Edmonton, AB T5J 2N3
www.health.alberta.ca
phone: 780-427-1432 (Edmonton)
Toll-free in Alberta: 310-0000,
then 780-427-1432

British Columbia Ministry
of Health Services
1515 Blanshard St.
Victoria, BC V8W 3C8
www.gov.bc.ca/health
phone: 250-387-6121 (Victoria)
604-660-2421 (Vancouver)
Toll-free in BC: 1-800-465-4911

Manitoba Health
300 Carlton St., Winnipeg, MB R3B 3M9
www.manitoba.ca/health
phone: toll-free: 1-800-392-1207

New Brunswick Department of Health
Box 5100, Fredericton, NB E3B 5G8
www.gnb.ca/0051/index-e.asp
Phone: 506-457-4800
Email: medicare@gnb.ca

Newfoundland and Labrador Department
of Health and Community Services
Confederation Building
Box 8700, St. John's, NL A1B 4J6
www.gov.nl.ca/health
Phone: 709-729-5021
Email: healthinfo@gov.nl.ca

Northwest Territories Department of
Health and Social Services
Box 1320, Yellowknife NT X1A 2L9
www.hlthss.gov.nt.ca
Phone: toll-free:
1-800-661-0830 or 1-867-777-7413
Email: hsa@gov.nt.ca

Nova Scotia Department of
Health and Wellness
Box 488, Halifax, NS B3J 2R8
Street address:
Joseph Howe Building
1690 Hollis St., Halifax, NS
www.gov.ns.ca/health/
Phone: 902-424-5818
Toll-free in Nova Scotia: 1-800-387-6665
TTY/TDD: 1-800-670-8888

Nunavut Department of
Health and Social Services
Box 1000, Station 1000
Iqaluit, NU X0A 0H0
www.gov.nu.ca/health/
Phone: 1-867-975-6000
Toll free: 1-867-975-5700
Email: info@gov.nu.ca

Ontario Ministry of
Health and Long-Term Care
10th Floor, Hepburn Block
80 Grosvenor St.
Toronto, ON M7A 1R3
www.health.gov.on.ca
Phone: general inquiries: 416-327-4327
Toll Free: 800-268-1153
TTY Toll Free: 800-387-5559

Prince Edward Island Department
of Health and Wellness
Box 2000
Charlottetown, PE C1A 7N8
www.gov.pe.ca/health
Phone: 902-368-6414
Fax: 902-368-4121

Quebec Ministry of Health
and Social Services
1075 Sainte-Foy Rd.
Québec, QC G1S 2M1
www.msss.gouv.qc.ca
Phone: 418-266-7005

Saskatchewan Health
3475 Albert St.
Regina, SK S4S 6X6
www.health.gov.sk.ca
Phone: 306-787-0146
Toll-free in Saskatchewan: 1-800-667-7766
Email: info@health.gov.sk.ca

Yukon Health and Social Services
Box 2703
Financial Plaza
Whitehorse, YT Y1A 2C6
www.hss.gov.yk.ca/
Phone: toll-free: 1-867-667-5209
Email: hss@gov.yk.ca

OTHER ORGANIZATIONS

CANADA

List of Canadian Children's Hospitals
http://www.aboutkidshealth.ca/En/HealthAZ/
TestsAndTreatments/Resources/Pages/Childrens-
Hospitals-in-Canada.aspx

**Canadian Foundation for
Women's Health**
780 Echo Dr.
Ottawa, ON K1S 5R7
http://www.cfwh.org/
Phone: 613.730.4192
Fax: 613.730.4314
Email: info@cfwh.org

Canadian Haemophilia Society
National Office
1255 University St., Ste. 400
Montreal, QC H3B 3B6
http://www.hemophilia.ca/
Phone: 514-848-0503
Toll-free: 1-800-668-2686
Fax: 514-848-9661
Email: chs@hemophilia.ca

**Canadian Institute for
Health Information**
495 Richmond Rd., Ste. 600
Ottawa, ON K2A 4H6
http://secure.cihi.ca/cihiweb/home_e.html
Fax: 613-241-8120

Canadian Medical Association
1867 Alta Vista Dr.
Ottawa, ON K1G 5W8
http://www.cma.ca/
Phone: toll free: 1-888-855-2555
Fax: 613-236-8864
Email: cmamsc@cma.ca

Canadian Women's Health Network
419 Graham Ave., Ste. 203
Winnipeg, MB R3C 0M3
http://www.cwhn.ca/en
Phone: 204-942-5500
Toll free: 1-888-818-9172
Fax: 204-989-2355
Email: cwhn@cwhn.ca

Children's Hospital of Eastern Ontario
401 Smyth Rd.
Ottawa, ON K1H 8L1
http://www.cheo.on.ca/en/contactcheo
Phone: 613-737-7600
Email: kouri@cheo.on.ca

Endometriosis Network
790 Bay St., 8th floor
Toronto, ON M5G 1N8
http://www.endometriosisnetwork.ca/
Email: info@endometriosisnetwork.ca

Fraser Institute
4th Floor, 1770 Burrard St.
Vancouver, BC V6J 3G7
http://www.fraserinstitute.org/
Phone: 604-688-0221
Fax: 604-688-8539

**The Hospital for Sick Children
Paediatric Gynaecology Clinic**
555 Unviersity Ave.
7th Floor, Black Wing
Toronto, ON M5G 1X8
http://www.sickkids.ca/gynaecology/
Phone: 416-813-6189
Fax: 416-613 -6192
Email: zarine.tilak@sickkids.ca

IWK Health Centre
Main IWK site and mailing address for all IWK
locations:
5850/5980 University Ave.
Box 9700
Halifax, NS B3K 6R8
http://www.iwk.nshealth.ca/index.
cfm?objectid=B2B9F409-D291-878D-
1A6F8F89710FDC83
Phone: 1-902-470-8888
Email: feedback@iwk.nshealth.ca

Mature Women's Centre
Victoria General Hospital, 3 North
2340 Pembina Highway
Winnipeg, MB R3T 2E8
http://www.vgh.mb.ca/mwc/halt.html
Phone: 204-477-3505
Fax: 204-275-0919
Email: info@maturewomenscentre.ca

Mowat Centre for Policy Information
School of Public Policy and Governance
University of Toronto
14 Queen's Park Cres. W., Room 61A
Toronto, ON M5S 3K9
Phone: 416-978-7857
Fax: 416-978-5079
Email: matthew@mowatcentre.ca

Society of Minimally
Invasive Gynecology
www.sogc.org/smig/index_e.aspx

Society of Obstetricians
and Gynecologists of Canada
780 Echo Dr.
Ottawa, ON K1S 5R7
http://www.sogc.org/index_e.asp
Phone: 613-730-4192
Toll-free: 1-800-561-2416
Fax: 613-730-4314
Email: helpdesk@sogc.com

UNITED STATES AND INTERNATIONAL

Association of American
Gynecological Laparoscopists
6757 Katella Ave.
Cypress, CA 90630-5105
www.aagl.org/
Phone: 714-503-6200
toll-free: 1-800-554-AAGL (2245)

Endometriosis Foundation of America
872 Fifth Ave.
New York, NY 10065
http://www.endofound.org/
Phone: 212-988-4160

Focused Ultrasound Surgery Foundation
1230 Cedars Court, Ste. F
Charlottesville, VA 22903
http://www.fusfoundation.org/
www.fibroidrelief.org
www.facebook.com/fibroidrelief
Phone: 434-220-4993

Hers Foundation
422 Bryn Mawr Ave.
Bala Cynwyd, PA 19004
http://www.hersfoundation.com/
Phone: 610-667-7757
Toll Free: 888-750-HERS (4377)
Fax: 610-667-8096
Email: hersfdn@earthlink.net

Hope for Fibroids, Inc.
www.hopeforfibroids.com

HysterSisters
http://www.hystersisters.com/

National Uterine Fibroid Foundation
Box 9688
Colorado Springs, CO 80932-0688
http://www.nuff.org/
Phone: 719.633.3454
Email: info@NUFF.org

World Endometriosis Research Foundation
www.endometriosisfoundation.org
www.endometriosis.org

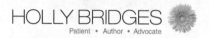

The
UNHysterectomy

HOLLY BRIDGES
Patient • Author • Advocate

Book Order Form

The UNHysterectomy is for every woman touched by the emotional, mental, physical and financial strain of painful, heavy menstrual bleeding. It's insightful, informative and empowering—a must-read for any woman looking to explore her options. Do you know a woman who could benefit? Or a doctor's office, hair salon or other venue that should have one or several on display?

Please send me _____ copies of the book *The UNHysterectomy* at $24.95 USD/CDN each.

I have enclosed a check payable to Holly Bridges Communications in the amount of $_____.

Full name: _____

Mailing address: _____

City: _____   State/Province: _____

Zip Code/Postal Code: _____   Telephone: _____

Email: _____

Free Shipping & Handling. Books are $24.95 each. HST will be added to book(s) shipped to Canada. Volume discount available for orders of 10 or more. Visit www.unhysterectomy.com for bulk rates.

Print, complete and mail with check to:
Holly Bridges Communications
1619 Orleans Blvd.
P.O. Box 58016 ORLEANS GARDEN
Ottawa, ON K1C 7E2

Order online at:
www.unhysterectomy.com

Send an email to:
sales@unhysterectomy.com